LOW CARB DIETS

EASY & HEALTHY WEIGHT LOSS PROGRAMS THAT REALLY WORK!

Susan Somerset Webb

LowCarb LifeStyles

It must be remembered that there is nothing
more difficult to plan, more doubtful of success,
nor more dangerous to manage
than the creation of a new system.
For the initiator has the enmity
of all who would profit by the preservation
of the old institution and
merely lukewarm defenders in those
who would gain by the new ones.

—Niccolo Machiavelli

TABLE OF CONTENTS

Introduction Why You Should Read This Book   1

Chapter 1 A Brief History of Dieting   5

Chapter 2 The Price We Pay   10

Chapter 3 All About Carbohydrates   14

Chapter 4 Eating Fat Does Not Make You Fat   22

Chapter 5 Beginning the Low Carb Lifestyle   33

Chapter 6 The Healthy Low Carb Lifestyle   42

Chapter 7 Four Groundbreaking Low Carb Diet
          Books Reviewed   50
Dr Atkins New Diet Revolution   50
The *Carbohydrate Addict's Lifespan Program*™   55
Protein Power   58
Sugar Busters!™   62

Chapter 8 Seven More Effective Low Carb Diet
          Books Reviewed   65
NeanderThin   65
Dr. Tony Perrone's Body-fat Breakthru   67
The Schwarzbein Principle   69
Eat Fat, Lose Weight   70
Charles Hunt's Diet Evolution™   70
Starch Madness   71
The Ketogenic Diet   72

Chapter 9 Three "Almost Low Carb Diet Books" Reviewed   74
The Zone   74
40-30-30 / Fat Burning Nutrition   76
The Low Carb Cookbook   78

Appendix A Foods Allowed on Six Different Diet Plans   81
Appendix B Questions and Answers   82

Bibliography and Resources   88

Why You Should Read This Book

We made a lot of wrong mistakes.

—Yogi Berra

America is the most food-abundant nation in the world. Food is plentiful, cheap and varied, and we don't even have to know how to cook to get it. In urban areas we can patronize restaurants that cater to our every culinary whim, from Mexican to Szechwan. And in small-town America, fast-food franchises seem to spring out from behind every corner. At home, those of us who do cook can watch the Food Channel, where 24-hours-a-day cooking experts tell us how to prepare everything from souffles to nuts. Americans have more food choices than any other society ever has had before.

This easy access to a cheap and plentiful food supply is making us fat. How fat? According to the National Heart, Lung and Blood Institute (NHLBI), by 1998 55 percent of Americans were overweight. Furthermore, if more than half the U.S. population can be considered overweight, NHLBI says that fully one-third of the adult population should be considered not just overweight but *obese.*

U.S. Health officials have long recognized that excess weight causes health problems. The United States Department of Agriculture (USDA), in an effort to curb our population's growing obesity,

1

instituted guidelines for a national low fat, low cholesterol, high carbohydrate diet. The visual aid for this diet was called the "food pyramid," and it was widely promoted.

Years later, with a substantial increase in the number of overweight Americans, we need to admit that this diet has failed for most of us. No matter how hard overweight Americans try to adhere to the USDA guidelines, they are still getting fat. This simple fact has drawn the attention of many researchers over the past two decades. They have tried to determine what it is about the average low fat, high carbohydrate diet that isn't producing the desired result.

Many of these same researchers also noticed that not only were Americans packing on unwanted pounds but the incidence of autoimmune system disorders such as diabetes and arthritis had greatly increased. According to the National Center for Health Statistics, overweight and obese adults have a much greater risk of contracting these diseases. The connection between the rise of these diseases and the implementation of USDA dietary guidelines cannot be ignored.

Could it be that diets just don't work? How many of you have had even a moderate amount of success staying on a diet? Have you lost weight and kept it off? Most experts agree that fewer than 10% of you are successful at maintaining weight loss.

It's important to understand that a low carbohydrate diet isn't just another diet plan that you grudgingly adhere to, lose your desired weight and then return to your old eating habits. This is a way of eating, not a diet! You will find that maintaining a low carb lifestyle is easy and rewarding. You'll not only lose weight, chances are you'll have more energy, reduce or eliminate your mood swings, and improve your health.

By choosing a low carb lifestyle you will be placing responsibility for your health right where it belongs—in your own hands. Making the proper food choices is empowering. Reading this and perhaps several of the very important books discussed further on will, hopefully, cause you to start asking questions about the way you have been eating.

Knowledge is indeed power.

In recent years a variety of diets higher in protein and fat and lower in carbohydrates have become popular. These are known as low carbohydrate (low carb) diets. Although surrounded by controversy these diets have a tremendous following. Not only have low carb dieters been successful in losing unwanted pounds, they have also kept those pounds off.

This book is intended as a resource for those people interested in learning about the benefits of restricting their carbohydrate intake. There are no new revelations or scientific facts presented here. This book is simply meant as an aid for those who have not yet decided exactly which low carb eating plan is right for them. Reviews of well-known and less well-known low carb diet books can be found beginning in chapter 7. But—please don't skip to that chapter immediately. Read each chapter in sequence so that you are able to make an informed decision about which diet is just right for you.

This book is very personal. I had been a successful vegetarian for several years and existed on carefully prepared pasta dishes with loads of salads. Fruit was breakfast and/or lunch. I had my fair share of bread. Toast for breakfast, veggie sandwich for lunch and fresh French bread with pasta nearly every evening. Bags of low fat potato chips or pretzels would sit on my desk as a reminder of how well I thought I was eating. Then there was the driving force behind my everyday existence—chocolate chip cookies. When these weren't available I'd settle for something less ethereal like pie, cake or ice cream. It really didn't matter. I was addicted.

In 1997 I was diagnosed with low blood sugar. I had conveniently ignored all the symptoms for years. Being tired and dizzy with constant mood swings and sugar cravings was a fact of life for me. After all, I was 50 and assumed it was all part of the female aging process. Also my waistline had expanded to the point that I no longer tucked in my shirts. I was thankful that black tights and big shirts were considered stylish. Stretch jeans were my saving grace.

While driving to a friend's on a very hot summer day, not having eaten anything but a banana, my body started to betray me. First, my hands and feet started to tingle, then my lips became numb. After that I noticed a roar in my ears and my vision became blurred. It didn't take me long to figure out that I was behind the wheel of a car travelling 50 miles an hour and losing conscienceness. After years of being ignored, my body finally had my full attention.

I was lucky, I escaped injury. But the experience was a wakeup call. After the diagnosis I began researching low blood sugar and its related illnesses. It quickly became clear to me that I was doing everything wrong in the food department. After even more research I became a low carbohydrate convert never to look back. Not only did I start to feel better almost immediately but I began to lose those few pesky unwanted pounds. What a bonus!

I soon became a rabid low carb evangelist. I wouldn't let my family and friends ignore me. I took every opportunity to try to convert them all. Most of them listened and have lost pounds as well as improved various health problems. The better I felt, the more pounds my friends shed, the more I wanted to know exactly how low carbohydrate plans worked. This book is the product of that search.

Be prepared to have a change of mind and heart about the way you eat. Use the resources at the end of this book to do your own research. Ask questions, be curious. But whatever you do, don't just cast aside the ideas presented here as the insane ramblings of a few crackpots. There is too much science to ignore.

CHAPTER 1

A Brief History of Dieting

THE HUNTER-GATHERER

In the spring of 1999, NBC's *Dateline* conducted a brief interview with Loren Cordain, Ph.D., an exercise physiology professor at Colorado State University. In the interview, Cordain explained why he felt we have been on the wrong dietary track for thousands of years. He said that we are genetically almost the same as our Stone Age ancestors of 40,000 years ago. Cordain believes that a Stone Age (or Paleolithic) diet can provide us with a basis from which to establish a contemporary diet.

Another researcher agrees. Dr. S. Boyd Eaton, a radiologist and medical anthropologist at Emory University, is considered an authority on Paleolithic diets. He believes that 99 percent of our genetic makeup dates from about 40,000 years ago and that 99.99 percent was formed about 10,000 years ago, before humans grew crops and domesticated animals for meat and milk.

What did our hunter-gatherer ancestors eat? Just as the term implies, they ate what they could kill or find. Primarily they ate meat from wild game, birds and fish. And they ate fruits, berries, vegetables, roots, nuts and eggs when they were in season and available. Their diet was high in protein with moderate fat content.

Our ancient ancestors were not obese. Furthermore, they did not appear to suffer from diseases like arthritis and diabetes. Nor, it seems, did they experience high blood pressure, elevated cholesterol or heart disease.

About 10,000 years ago (the beginning of the Neolithic period), the advent of agriculture dramatically changed the hunter-gatherer's diet. The cultivation of grains and domestic livestock probably evolved because it was easier than taking up a sharp stick and searching for game, perhaps for days. Food cultivation provided a dependable and constantly available source of nutrition.

However, along with the radical changes made by our Neolithic ancestors in the way they lived, there came a change in their general health. The digestive system that worked so wonderfully for over two million years was suddenly required to process food that it hadn't ever before encountered. Our digestive tract evolved to process meat, fat, and high-fiber carbohydrates (fruits, vegetables, berries, etc.). It was not designed to process the refined carbohydrates (breads, cereals, and sugar, etc.) that our Neolithic ancestors introduced to their diet.

The skeletal remains of Neolithic (agricultural) humans differ significantly from those of the preceding Paleolithic era. Archeologists have found that human remains of the Neolithic era show signs of malnutrition: rotting teeth and brittle bones. These conditions are not found in the remains of the Paleolithic hunter-gatherer. The implication is that the introduction of cultivated foods brought with it a deterioration in overall physical well-being.

THE INDUSTRIAL REVOLUTION

Although enormous improvements in food and animal cultivation occurred over the centuries, the basic changes to the human diet made by our Neolithic ancestors remained in place until the beginning of the 19th century. With the advent of the Industrial Revolution there was a population exodus from rural farms to urban factories. In order to feed the increased urban population new food production methods were devised.

Scientists have concluded that although our diets have changed radically in the last 10,000 years, our digestive systems are essentially no different than those of our prehistoric ancestors.

Commercially produced foods became popular because they were cheap to make and kept well. White flour—stripped of its nutrients in processing—could be stored for longer periods of time than whole wheat grain or, for that matter, fresh fruits and vegetables. Also at this time, sugar became a household staple. Soon after these drastic changes were introduced to our diet, there was a dramatic increase in the incidence of obesity and many immune system diseases such as arthritis, diabetes and heart disease.

In the mid-19th century, English businessman William Banting was one of many people to express concern over his expanding waistline. After consulting with several medical advisors the obese Banting was luckily referred to someone who suggested he abstain from ". . . Bread, butter, milk, sugar, beer, and potatoes. . . ." So successful was he in reducing his weight that in 1864 he wrote and published a pamphlet outlining those principles that he felt were necessary for a long, healthy and fit life.

Of all the parasites that affect humanity I do not know of, nor can I imagine, any more distressing than that of Obesity, and having just emerged from a very long probation in this affliction, I am desirous of circulating my humble knowledge and experience for the benefit of my fellow man, with an earnest hope it may lead to the same comfort and happiness I now feel under the extraordinary change—which might almost be termed miraculous had it not been accomplished by the most simple common sense-means.

Thus begins Mr. Banting's intriguing *Letter On Corpulence*, a discussion of what today most people would characterize as a low carbohydrate diet. Although Banting's ideas were effective they did not create enough interest to have a significant effect on the overweight population of his time. Obesity continued to be a problem.

Following closely on the heels of Banting came several other self-proclaimed dietary experts, one of whom was Dr. John Harvey Kellogg. In an effort to address the mounting number of health complaints as well as the increase in obesity, Kellogg opened a health resort in Battle Creek, Michigan in the late 1800s.

In direct opposition to Mr. Banting's recommendations for a healthful life, Dr. Kellogg advocated a high carbohydrate, low fat diet with an emphasis on breakfast cereals and other food items that he himself developed. Meat was prohibited. Although many of Dr. Kellogg's patients were successful at losing considerable weight, they were forced to return to him again and again because they, like most dieters today, could not keep off the unwanted pounds. Despite his mixed success, Kellogg's ideas about diet and nutrition can be considered a precursor to the USDA food pyramid.

MODERN IDEAS

Fast forward to the 1960s, the decade that spawned the proliferation of fast-food restaurants. Ideally suited to a generation that claimed it didn't have time to sit down for a home-cooked meal, fast food has become synonymous with the American way of life. It has become all too easy to take a detour through the drive-thru for fries and a shake on the way to your next appointment. Not to have done this at one time or another makes you practically un-American.

Fast forward again. In the December 12, 1981 issue of the medical journal *The Lancet,* the results of a five-year study were published. This study followed a group of Norwegian men thought to be at greater risk of heart disease because they all smoked and had high total cholesterol levels. Divided into two groups, one half was told they should continue their current diet and behaviors. The other group was given advice about a more healthy lifestyle that included better eating habits and reduced drinking and smoking.

The results were astounding. The men in the group that had altered their lifestyles had decreased their heart disease and death by 47 percent over the group that made no changes. Their total cholesterol levels had dropped dramatically.

This good news was unfortunately misinterpreted. The men in the group that changed lifestyles had reduced their smoking by 45 percent. At that time it was not known that smoking increased cholesterol numbers. Consequently, it was assumed that the decrease in dietary fat and cholesterol had been responsible for the 47 percent reduction in heart disease and death. The misinterpretation of this data may have spawned the low fat movement. Dr. Diana Schwarzbein discusses this subject in detail in her excellent and informative 1999 book *The Schwarzbein Principle*. (See chapter 8 for a review of *The Schwarzbein Principle*.)

Still, the controversy rages. There seem to be as many opinions as to why we are a nation of obese and unhealthy people as there are ways to lose those pounds. Medical anthropologist S. Boyd Eaton believes America's obesity problem is because our genetic makeup has not been able to keep up with the enormous dietary changes made in the last 10,000 years. We are putting 20th century foods into bodies that haven't changed genetically for thousands and thousands of years.

The Price We Pay

BEING OVERWEIGHT IS AN EXPENSIVE BUSINESS

Epidemologists at Harvard University have estimated that treating obesity and its related diseases—high blood pressure, heart disease and diabetes—cost the American public (conservatively) $45.8 billion in 1990. This doesn't take into account time spent away from work which adds $23 billion. Then add another $33 billion for weight-loss products and services. *The staggering total cost per year (in 1990) is over $101.8 billion.*

The Diet Industry

Diet industries have sprung up everywhere to take advantage of the upward swing in obesity. Diet drinks that supplement or substitute for meals have become popular. We have come to believe that if the label says "nutritionally complete" we can assume it must be good for us. Commercials for some of these products might make seniors believe that a meal in a can will keep you trim and young at heart as well.

The newest diet drug, fat absorber, nutritional supplement, diet clinic or weight loss program is always just around the corner. Television infomercials for a multitude of exercise equipment are on at every hour of every day. And, let's not forget the pharmaceutical industry. Remember Fen-Phen? The American

> *The Institute of Medicine defines the dramatic increase in health care costs related to obesity as an epidemic. Obesity kills 300,000 Americans a year.*

public was convinced the best way to lose weight was to take a pill and just keep on eating.

The Hidden Price of Low Fat Products

More than just a few corporations benefit from obesity and its related diseases. You don't have to walk too far into your local supermarket before you begin to notice the huge array of diet-oriented products. Most of them, labeled low fat and/or sugar free, are promoted with the implication that you can consume them without concern for your weight.

What these food manufacturers don't tell you is that because of the trend toward low fat, many of them have disguised the loss of fat with the addition of high-fructose corn syrup. High-fructose corn syrup is a high-calorie sweetener, and several researchers believe that it is even worse for your body than sugar.

Sugar is a carbohydrate. So, in essence, most of the low fat products that line supermarket shelves are loaded with carbohydrates. As you will learn later, it is these carbohydrates that are keeping America fat.

It is estimated that every American consumes an average of over 150 pounds of sugar annually. If you think about that for a moment, you will realize that your consumption of all this sugar is a major factor in your struggle with excess weight. Unfortunately, most of us are unaware that we are consuming sugar in the guise of high-fructose corn syrup and other sugar derivatives present in many of the foods we eat every day.

While most of us are aware of how sugar contributes to obesity, the other dangers of sugar are less well-known. According to Drs. E. Cheraskin and W. M. Ringsdorf (*Psychodietetics*, 1989) sugar plays a major role in the development of many illnesses including kidney stones, cardiovascular disease and intestinal cancer. They also believe there is a prominent connection between sugar and mental illness. Dr. Diana Schwarzbein, founder of The Endocrinology Institute of Santa Barbara, believes that sugar was the cause of many of her childhood illnesses such as acne, asthma and irritable bowel syndrome.

Syndrome X, another lesser-known yet deadly disease, is effected by carbohydrates (sugar). Syndrome X is the name of a group of risk factors for heart disease associated with insulin resistance. An estimated 90,000 adult Americans are at risk of this often lethal disease. As you will learn later on, over-consumption of carbohydrates is directly related to insulin resistance.

William Dufty takes over 200 pages to describe the evils of sugar and its derivatives in his groundbreaking 1975 book *Sugar Blues*. Nearly all the diet plans reviewed in this book talk about the negative impact of sugar. So we must ask ourselves why we continue to consume foods that have substituted fructose, sucrose or sugar for fat. Clearly such substitutions are at the expense of our health.

THE SOCIAL CONSEQUENCES

Almost as important as the health issues are the social and mental health consequences of excess poundage. Even though nearly 55 percent of us are overweight, you will rarely see overweight people on television or in the movies. Virtually all media project an image of a trim, athletic body that is not in sync with reality. Consequently, those of us who are overweight are made to feel abnormal or inferior.

More significantly, the overweight are less likely to advance in their careers as fast (or as far) as their slimmer peers. Getting hired for a new job is more difficult too, no matter how qualified you are.

*Even the diet and energy bars at health
food stores can be loaded with sugar or its
derivatives.*

The list of disadvantages seems endless. If you are severely overweight, you may not be able to shop for your clothes at regular retail stores. You certainly won't be able to fit in a economy car, or squeeze into a coach class airline seat. You may find it difficult to make new friends, and it's darn near impossible to meet Mr. or Ms. Right. Overweight people are prone to depression and withdrawal from society. Many find their only comfort by eating more and more food.

CHAPTER 3

All About Carbohydrates

THE BASICS

The food we eat is divided into three groups or elements. These elements are protein, fat and carbohydrate. When you consume carbohydrates your body processes them just like it would process sugar. Because your body recognizes all carbohydrates the same way, a bowl of white rice is processed virtually the same way as a piece of chocolate cake. Sort of makes you stop and think about all those rice cakes we've been told are so good for us, doesn't it?

If you are like most Americans you have tried to be good at following the United States Department of Agriculture (USDA) Food Guide Pyramid (see Figure 1). The Food Guide Pyramid is a tool developed by the USDA. It illustrates a properly balanced diet, according to the USDA's current thinking on nutritional health. If you've been following these guidelines, 75–85 percent of your daily food consumption has been in the form of carbohydrates.

All carbohydrates—grains, vegetables, fruit and sugar—are recognized and processed by your body in virtually the same way.

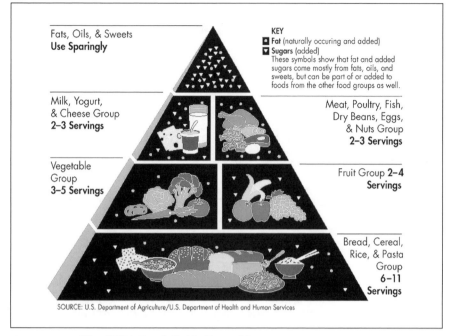

Figure 1.   The USDA Food Guide Pyramid

A typical breakfast that follows the USDA Food Guide Pyramid might look something like this.

Orange juice	22 carbohydrate grams
Toast with margarine	20 carbohydrate grams
Low fat cereal	35 carbohydrate grams
Banana	26 carbohydrate grams
Skim milk	12 carbohydrate grams

The high carbohydrate content of this breakfast (a total of 115 grams) causes your body to identify and process everything you just ate as if it were sugar.

Insulin and Your Waistline

We all need energy to live. This energy is provided in the form of food. The three elements—carbohydrate, protein and fat—provide

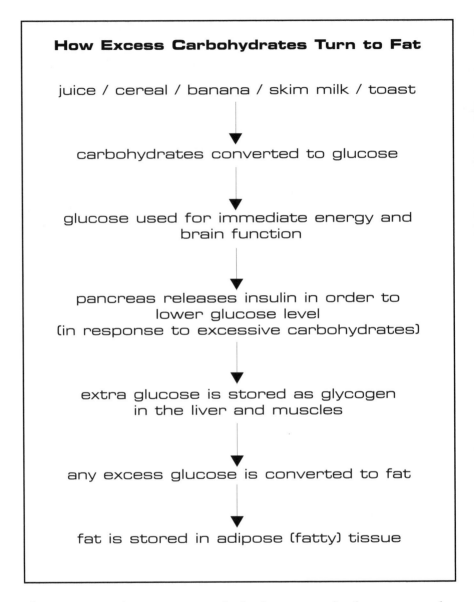

How Excess Carbohydrates Turn to Fat

juice / cereal / banana / skim milk / toast

↓

carbohydrates converted to glucose

↓

glucose used for immediate energy and brain function

↓

pancreas releases insulin in order to lower glucose level
(in response to excessive carbohydrates)

↓

extra glucose is stored as glycogen in the liver and muscles

↓

any excess glucose is converted to fat

↓

fat is stored in adipose (fatty) tissue

that energy. When we eat carbohydrates our body converts the sugar (remember, the body recognizes carbohydrates as sugar) into glucose. Glucose is used by the muscles as energy for motion. Glucose is also necessary for brain function.

When too many carbohydrates are consumed, such as in the breakfast above, there is an excess of glucose (sugar). The body efficiently converts all of this extra glucose into glycogen. The glycogen is then stored in the liver for future use by the brain.

(Remember, the brain needs glucose to function.) Glycogen is also stored in the muscles for immediate energy (where it cannot be accessed by the brain). The muscles and liver have a limited capacity for glycogen storage. When that capacity is reached the pancreas instructs the body to convert all extra glycogen into fat to be stored in fatty tissues.

The pancreas has many functions. One of its most important functions is the production of the powerful hormone called insulin. The pancreas releases insulin into the blood to help regulate (lower) blood sugar.

A few hours after your cereal, toast and juice breakfast you might begin to feel "foggy." Unless you ran a marathon, the 115 grams of carbohydrates you consumed was more than you needed. The excess carbohydrates caused your blood sugar to rise. Your pancreas then sent out enough insulin to lower your excess blood sugar (glucose) that was caused by all the carbohydrates. This insulin surge dramatically lowers your blood sugar level and causes you to have that foggy feeling. Remember—your brain needs glucose to function.

Hypoglycemia

Hypoglycemia is really just another word for low blood sugar. People with this condition experience a radical drop in blood sugar after eating a carbohydrate-rich meal. It is a medical condition that can exhibit many psychological and physical symptoms. These symptoms include:

PSYCHOLOGICAL	PHYSICAL
Confusion	Fainting or blackouts
Restlessness	Blurred vision
Antisocial behavior	Shakiness/tremors
Depression	Indigestion
Anxiety	Joint pain
Difficulty in concentration	Exhaustion
Irritability	Headache

Carlton Fredericks, PhD., (*New Low Blood Sugar and You*, 1985) believes that low blood sugar can cause adverse psychiatric symptoms in an otherwise mentally stable person. He also suggests that it can cause alcoholism and in some cases can lead to drug addiction. Difficult to detect, low blood sugar can go untreated for years, exhibiting many of the symptoms listed above.

Hyperinsulimia

The more carbohydrate-rich food someone with hypoglycemia eats, the more the pancreas responds with greater and greater amounts of insulin. After years of abuse the pancreas becomes extremely sensitive to even a small rise in blood sugar. So sensitive, in fact, that it may eventually be tricked into releasing insulin without your eating any carbohydrates at all. Sitting in a restaurant looking at a menu or smelling food being prepared may be enough to cause a sensitive pancreas to release insulin.

Because the production of excess insulin causes your body to store fat, your body becomes a fat-storing machine.

When the pancreas becomes hypersensitive and begins to overproduce insulin this condition is called hyperinsulimia or insulin resistance. Some researchers have found that nearly 75 percent of overweight Americans suffer from insulin resistance. One physical sign of this condition is fat stored around the stomach or midsection. This is primarily where excess glucose is stored (as fat) in someone with insulin resistance. Someone with hyperinsulimia may very well have thin arms and legs but will carry all their excess weight around the middle.

If this condition is allowed to continue undiagnosed and untreated, hyperinsulimia (insulin resistance) can result in Type II diabetes. According to the American Diabetes Association, diabetes is the third leading cause of death in the United States. Of the eight million diagnosed diabetics, 95 percent have what is known as Type II diabetes, or insulin-resistant diabetes. Nearly a quarter of Americans between the ages of 65 and 74 have Type II diabetes. The cost of treating this prevalent disease is a staggering $92 billion per year. (This figure includes not only treatment costs but loss of productivity.)

Dr. Richard K. Bernstein, in *Dr. Bernstein's Diabetes Solution*, talks about Type II diabetes and the fact that it often goes undiagnosed. He refers to it as the silent killer. According to Bernstein, this is because the symptoms are easy to miss. Often Type II is discovered through one of its complications such as hypertension or vision trouble.

TYPE II DIABETES SYMPTOMS
Frequent urination
Blurred vision
Slow-healing skin infections

YOUR NEW BEST FRIEND, GLUCAGON

Now that we have a pretty good idea of what it is that insulin does —causes our bodies to store fat—we need to examine how these fat stores are accessed and used for energy.

Glucagon is another hormone secreted by the pancreas. It is insulin's exact opposite. Released by dietary protein, it is responsible for releasing stored glucose (sugar) from the liver for energy. It also helps maintain proper brain function and is responsible for telling the fat cells to release stored fat for use as energy.

Remember, excess glucose is stored in the liver and muscles, and what is not used there is stored as fat. Assuming once again that you had a bowl of cereal with banana, toast and juice at breakfast, not only do your insulin levels rise, but glucagon is suppressed. This process prevents any stored fat from being burned.

Many researchers speculate that we have an evolutionary predisposition to the storage of food energy—or glucose—as fat. Although they are not sure exactly why this happens, they have some theories. Some suggest that our prehistoric ancestors, unsure when they would get their next meal, survived because their bodies stored food energy (fat) to be used when food was

Glucagon releases glucose stored as fat.

An excess of insulin (a result of eating too many carbohydrates) suppresses the release of glucagon.

scarce. Since we are 99.99 percent genetically identical to our ancient ancestors this would mean that we too are programmed to store food energy for later use. However, since we live in a nation of such incredible abundance it seems unlikely that many of us will have to worry about food the way Paleolithic humans did.

The body is a marvelously complex system and what has just been discussed here is a very simplified version of what happens when an excess of carbohydrate-rich foods is consumed. Most of the diet books reviewed in later chapters give a much more detailed account of this process and are good sources for more information.

A FEW WORDS ABOUT FIBER

As Martha Stewart might say about fiber: "It's a good thing." We all know fiber improves bowel function and helps to prevent constipation. What most of us aren't aware of is how fiber functions to stabilize blood sugar. It is believed that fiber slows the absorption of carbohydrates. It may also slow the pancreas' release of insulin in response to carbohydrates. This means that eating a whole orange (which means consuming the juice *and* the fiber) is better for you than drinking a glass of orange juice. The pulp (fiber) of the orange helps slow down the production of insulin.

Some researchers believe that the fruit and vegetable juicing we have been told is so good for us has actually done a few things that aren't so good. Because juicing removes the fiber from fruits and vegetables there is nothing to help slow down the insulin response. Consequently, there is a rapid rise in glucose with a rapid release of insulin to control it. The result is low blood sugar as well as the inevitable storage of excess glucose as fat.

In *Protein Power*, Drs. Michael and Mary Dan Eades suggest that fiber doesn't act as a carbohydrate in your system. Therefore, they say, the usable carbohydrate content of a food is the gram weight of the carbohydrate *minus* the gram weight of its fiber. As an example, a piece of high fiber whole wheat bread might have 15 grams of carbohydrate. However, if you subtract the amount of its dietary fiber, which might be three grams, the total usable carbo-hydrate of that particular piece of bread would be only 12 grams.

Most—if not all—diet gurus agree that including fiber in your eating plan is very important. In fact, most believe that fiber is *essential* to the success of any low carbohydrate diet. The Eades recommend 25 grams of fiber daily.

CHAPTER 4

Eating Fat Does Not Make You Fat

An invasion of armies can be resisted, but not an idea whose time has come.

—Victor Hugo

Since the early 80s we have been told by the experts that if we eat fat we will gain weight. Remember the adage: "Fat past these lips is fat on these hips"? To avoid all that bad fat we have had to fill up in other ways. Consider the three food elements: protein, carbohydrate and fat. We've been told to eliminate—as much as possible— one whole group: fat. That leaves protein and carbohydrates. And, because most forms of protein contain some fat, a lot of people eliminated a lot of protein as well. That left carbohydrates. We were told that carbohydrates were not fattening. How could a rice cake cause us to put on unwanted pounds? As a result, many of us ate all the pasta, bread, potatoes, rice cakes, fruit and vegetables that we wanted.

We didn't believe that we could possibly gain weight by eating pasta, low-fat crackers, potatoes, fruit or rice because they don't contain fat. Remember, we were told that it was dietary fat that was making us fat. That led to the conclusion that we could even eat fat-free potato chips and muffins without adverse consequences.

Remember the breakfast discussed in chapter 3? It consisted of orange juice, toast, and cereal with skim milk and banana. Because we were striving for a low fat meal, this breakfast was made up of nearly all carbohydrates. Remember, carbohydrate consumption increases insulin production and insulin is the fat-storing hormone.

After eating such a breakfast, sometime before lunch you will begin to feel the effect of the carbohydrate-laden meal. Your brain will start to signal its need for glucose so that it can function properly. This "signal" is a pre-lunch foggy or sleepy feeling with which you may be familiar. It occurs because your pancreas had to produce an excessive amount of insulin in response to all those carbohydrates you had at breakfast. As a result, you may start to exhibit signs of low blood sugar.

We now know that most people consume very limited protein and fat when they are on a low fat diet. When that happens, the body is soon forced to use the proteins and fats that it has stored as lean muscle tissue. Since muscle tissue weighs more than fat, you lose weight. However, *you are losing muscle mass, not fat.*

It is important to understand that the more muscle mass you have the faster your rate of metabolism. The faster your metabolism, the better your fat-burning ability. When you lose muscle mass you diminish your ability to burn stored fat. By limiting dietary fat, you begin to lose this vital muscle tissue.

Eventually, after continued low fat, high carbohydrate eating, you may begin to see the signs of high insulin levels. In some cases one sign may be an increase in your waist size. Remember, people who are insulin resistant generally carry their excess weight around the stomach or midsection. You've probably noticed that there are certain people who have real difficulty losing their spare tire no matter what they do. This is often because a low fat diet produces large amounts of insulin. Insulin is the fat-storing hormone. And for those on long-term low-fat high-carbohydrate diets this extra fat is stored at their waistline.

Fat satisfies hunger. Known as the satiety nutrient, it is digested slowly and does, therefore, send signals to the brain that you are satisfied. Carbohydrates, on the other hand, pass through the stomach into the small intestine almost immediately and don't send the necessary "full" signals to the brain. This means that you are satisfied faster and for a longer period of time if you include fat in your diet.

It also means that you consume much less fat than carbohydrates. Did you ever notice how easy it is to overeat carbohydrates? Most of us could sit down and eat several chocolate chip cookies before we felt satisfied but try and eat the equivalent amount of cheese and see what happens. By eating a little fat throughout the day you can suppress hunger and also burn stored fat.

In his book *Dr. Bernstein's Diabetes Solution*, Dr. Richard K. Bernstein calls the way fat has been demonized as "the Big Fat Lie." He believes emphatically that Americans are overweight because of the pervasive myth that fat consumption is fattening.

So, what have you accomplished by eating a low-fat, high-carbohydrate diet? You've:

• Lost vital muscle mass
• Gained body fat
• Dramatically increased your insulin production

The result of all this low fat dieting has been less than favorable for a large percentage of Americans.

• 55 percent of all Americans are overweight.
• In 1997, according to the National Institutes of Health, there were 8 million diagnosed diabetics in the United States. That number increases annually by about 700,000.
• The incidence of immune system disorders such as heart disease, arthritis, and allergies has risen dramatically.

It hasn't been only because of our expanding waistlines that we've avoided fat. We've also been convinced that eating fat can cause serious damage to our hearts by clogging our blood vessels. According to many experts, the real truth about low fat diets has been available for years but has failed to reach the public because of an intensive media campaign promoting a low fat diet.

Some research has shown that it is only the combination of low fat with high fiber in a diet that produces lower blood fat levels,

Fat helps to unlock stored body fat

Fat maintains cell membranes

Fat stores hormones

Fat is used as energy

Fat acts as insulation

Fat aids nervous system function

Fat stabilizes joints and muscles

not low fat alone. However, Americans have very little interest in high fiber foods because, as a rule, they don't taste very good. It didn't take food manufacturers very long to realize that they couldn't sell high fiber foods. So instead they concentrated on producing tasty low fat products that often contained excessive amounts of sugar.

Extensive research done by scientists around the world provides clinical evidence that low fat diets generally have not been successful in producing weight loss and lowering blood fat levels. So, not only have low fat, high carbohydrate diets made us fatter, they have adversely effected our health.

A good example of how eating fat affects your body would be to look at the traditional diet of Eskimos. Several of the diet plans reviewed in this book talk about the Eskimo diet as a perfect example of how eating fat does not make you fat. Eskimo diets consist mainly of protein and large amounts of fat with very limited carbohydrates. During the arctic's winter carbohydrates are practically nonexistent.

Surprisingly, given this extraordinary diet, Eskimos have a very low incidence of heart disease, obesity and many other diseases associated with high insulin levels. This remarkable finding has been attributed not only to low carbohydrate consumption but to the fact that the Eskimos eat cold-water fish such as salmon, cod, trout, sardines, tuna and herring. These fish contain what are called omega-3 fatty acids—the "good" fat.

Arctic explorer, Vilhjalmar Stefansson, maintained an Eskimo diet for a year. At the end of the year he was not only thinner but he had lowered cholesterol levels as well.

In her book *Eat Fat, Lose Weight*, Ann Louise Gittleman discusses several recent low fat studies. One that is particularly interesting is the Nurses' Health Study published in the *New England Journal of Medicine*, November 1997. The study followed 80,000 nurses between the ages of 34 and 59 for 14 years. The remarkable results showed that what really matters healthwise is not the amount of fat consumed but the kind of fat.

THE GOOD FATS AND THE BAD FATS

For years you have been hearing that there are three kinds of fats: polyunsaturated, monounsaturated and saturated. In order to have a more clear understanding of what these terms mean, a very brief chemistry and Greek lesson is in order.

First the Greek. Poly means *many*, mono means *one* and un means *not*. So, polyunsaturated means *many not saturated*, monounsaturated means *one not saturated*, and unsaturated means *not saturated*. Most fats contain a proportion of each of these three basic types but are normally described according to which type predominates in their make up. Now on to the science part.

What the prefixes *mono, poly* and *un* refer to is how many hydrogen atoms each fat molecule holds. Saturated fats contain molecules that are completely saturated with hydrogen. These fats are normally solid at room temperature.

TABLE 4–1. EXAMPLES OF SATURATED FATS

animal fat	cocoa butter	margarine
butter	coconut oil	shortening
cheese	cream	sour cream

For nearly 20 years we have been avoiding these fats because we were told that they would make us fat, clog our arteries or even cause cancer. Now we understand that limited amounts of these fats are not only good for us, they are essential for maintaining a healthy body.

Polyunsaturated fat molecules are missing several hydrogen atoms. They are liquid at room temperature and when refrigerated. Remember the Eskimos? Some polyunsaturated fish oils that they consume contain an omega-3 fatty acid that has been shown to be effective in fighting both heart disease and cancer. It is important to note that these polyunsaturated oils should not be used for cooking as heat damages their structure. This been shown in laboratory tests to promote cancer.

TABLE 4–2. EXAMPLES OF POLYUNSATURATED FATS

corn oil	safflower oil	sunflower oil
cottonseed oil	salmon oil	wheat germ oil
flaxseed oil	sesame seed oil	

Monounsaturated fats are known as the good guys. They are liquid at room temperature but turn solid when refrigerated. Their chemical structure is not damaged when heated and these fats have been shown to lower cholesterol.

TABLE 4–3. EXAMPLES OF MONOUNSATURATED FATS

almond oil	fish oil	peanut oil
avocado oil	grapeseed oil	walnut oil
canola oil	olive oil	

Transfats

The butter vs. margarine battle has been raging for as long as we have been listening to the low fat gurus. It seems everyone but the French have been avoiding the proclaimed evils of butter. Americans were quick to embrace tubs of spreadable margarine because we were told it would help to keep our cholesterol in check.

However, it looks like the French had it right all along. Margarine belongs to a group of fats known as transfats. In transfats the fat molecules have been altered by the manufacturers so that the fat is more solid, easier to work with and has a longer shelf life. Transfats are not recognized by the body in the same way that natural fats are. These transformed fats are very bad for us because they are now saturated. Transfats have been proven to raise blood cholesterol levels. This is quite the reverse of what we have been told by the health industry for the last two decades.

The other side of the coin is butter. Butter, unlike vegetable oil, from which margarine is made, is solid at room temperature. Like animal fats and solid vegetable fats, butter has been demonized by low fat advocates. The truth about the benefits of butter are finally being revealed. Butter is rich in several essential vitamins and also selenium, an important antioxidant.

Should you want more detailed information about fats, several of the books reviewed in chapters 7 through 9 explore the subject in more detail. Especially good are *Eat Fat, Lose Weight* by Ann Louise Gittleman, and *The Schwarzbein Principle* by Diana Schwarzbein.

What About Cholesterol?

The authors of all of the diet plans reviewed in this book agree that dietary fat and cholesterol are a problem—but only if consumed with excess carbohydrates.

It is a normal function of the liver to produce cholesterol because we require it for good health. Cholesterol is an important part of cell structure. If you are deficient in cholesterol, cell structure is compromised. Unless you consume adequate amounts of dietary fat and cholesterol, your liver will produce its own choles-

Excess carbohydrates produce elevated insulin levels which, in turn, instruct your body to produce excess amounts of cholesterol.

terol to keep your cells healthy. However, through a biochemical reaction with carbohydrates, the liver begins to *over*produce cholesterol, making more than it needs. The only way to halt this process is by eating dietary cholesterol.

One of the major proponents of low carb diets, Dr. Robert Atkins, cites many scientific studies that confirm this. He is convinced that carbohydrate-restricted diets lower serum lipid levels (which include cholesterol).

THE IMPORTANCE OF PROTEIN

Because of the low fat movement, an essential part of our diet has been reduced or in some cases totally eliminated. Many forms of protein contain fat. Foods like red meat, eggs and even nuts have been targeted as practically evil by low fat advocates.

Protein is one of the three food elements; it is necessary for the constant rebuilding of cells in our bodies. Proteins support our immune system. Protein is also necessary for the production of hormones. Without sufficient protein, hormonal production becomes imbalanced. A lack of protein can also cause other symptoms such as malnutrition, dry skin, hair loss and depression. A protein-deficient diet will also cause water retention and bloating.

Twenty-two amino acids combine to make up protein. These amino acids build and repair muscle cells, connective tissue, skin and blood. Many of these amino acids can only be obtained through your diet. Proteins that provide all the essential amino acids are called complete proteins. Animal protein such as beef, poultry, fish and eggs are complete proteins. One ounce of animal protein contains seven grams of protein.

Most of the diet plans reviewed in this book suggest different protein requirements. One suggests 70–80 grams a day for men and 60–70 grams a day for women. Another plan suggests that protein should be 25 to 40 percent of your total food intake. Others have their own very specific way of calculating the daily amount of protein their plan requires for each individual and offer formulas to help calculate this specific amount. Despite their small differences it is interesting to note that all of the plans recommend much more protein than the 10 percent or so suggested by the USDA Food Guide Pyramid.

Proteins satisfy appetite quickly. They cause digestive enzymes to be produced in the stomach. These enzymes, together with the protein, cause the stomach to enlarge. This does two things: it signals the brain that food is coming and it also creates a feeling of fullness. These two facts are what keep humans (and animals) from overeating protein.

Carbohydrates do not produce the same effect. They do not make you feel full quickly because they go right through the stomach and into the small intestine where the digestion process begins. When you eat carbohydrates, enzymes are not produced in the stomach for digestion so the stomach does not become enlarged. Consequently, it takes longer for the brain to receive the message that food has arrived. Since it takes longer for the brain to receive the message we continue to eat carbohydrates long after we are actually full.

You will recall that the pancreas produces both insulin and glucagon. Insulin is a fat-storing hormone and glucagon releases stored fat for use as energy. When there is too much insulin present, glucagon is prevented from unlocking stored fat. In other words, not only will a well-balanced diet of protein, fat and carbohydrate prevent too much insulin from being produced, it is the key to unlocking stored fat.

According to Drs. Michael and Mary Dan Eades (authors of *Protein Power*) it is possible that 50 percent of the weight lost on

Protein is necessary for the rebuilding and repair of cells, muscle tissue, skin and blood

Protein is necessary for the production of hormones.

Proteins satisfy hunger faster than carbohydrates

Protein provides a steady flow of energy

Protein helps to stabilize blood sugar

Insufficient protein can cause malnutrition, dry skin, hair loss, depression, water retention and bloating.

a low-fat high-carbohydrate diet is lean muscle because protein has been restricted or even eliminated. The less lean muscle tissue you have the lower your metabolism, the less fat burned.

THE CONTROVERSIAL KETONES

As we now know, low fat diets are very high in carbohydrates and the body recognizes these carbohydrates as sugar. The body then converts that sugar into glucose and uses what it needs at the moment for energy. The remaining glucose is stored for later use in the liver and the *remainder of that* as fat. Insulin levels are also increased during this process. An increase in insulin levels not only causes fat to be stored but eventually causes symptoms of low blood sugar.

On a low carbohydrate diet the amount of glucose in your body is greatly diminished and insulin production is decreased. Because of the very limited amount of glucose in your system your body is forced to burn fat instead of glucose. When stored fat is burned it produces a by-product known as ketone bodies or ketones. These ketones are used for fuel by both your brain and body. Incompletely burned fat in the form of ketones is released from your body by your stool, urine and breath.

There are those who suggest that ketones can damage brain cells and do harm to kidneys. However, there is an abundance of scientific evidence to the contrary. But, note that all medical experts believe that ketosis is dangerous for diabetics.

This is a very simplified explanation of the ketosis process. For those of you who require more detail, pick up a copy of Lyle McDonald's book *The Ketogenic Diet* (reviewed in chapter 8). It has by far the most complete discussion of ketones and ketosis.

CHAPTER 5

Beginning the Low Carb Lifestyle

Never eat more than you can lift.

—Miss Piggy

HEALTH EVALUATION

Before beginning any new diet it's essential to have a baseline from which to gauge your progress. A baseline would include your weight (make sure you have a scale) and the state of your general health. Virtually all of the diet plan books that are reviewed in this book recommend—*at the very least*—a visit to your physician for a checkup. A number of books recommend various blood tests.

For a lot of us the process of getting standard blood tests every year or two is just a matter of course. However, there are many people who believe that having blood tests done is a waste of time and money unless they're sick.

All of the books reviewed in this book (chapters 7 through 9) have differing opinions about which medical tests they feel are essential before beginning their particular plans. These views range from no tests at all to a complete laboratory work-up.

There is no question that working with your physician is of primary importance when changing your diet or exercise regime. When you visit your physician, you may want to take this book (or another low carb diet book) with you. If your physician does not initially support a low carbohydrate eating plan, your chosen book may provide information to your doctor of which he or she was previously unaware.

CARBOHYDRATE AWARENESS

First of all, throw away all your old ideas about diet foods. Low carb diet plans include poultry, fish, shellfish, meat, fats/oils, dairy products (heavy cream, butter and some cheeses), nuts, most vegetables and some fruit. A couple of these diet plans even allow desserts! Depriving yourself of essential nutrients, like protein and fat, is a thing of the past.

The most important aspect of a low carb diet is counting carbohydrate grams. According to most low carb gurus, it is not necessary to count calories or fat grams or to restrict your food intake in any other way except limiting carbohydrates. *You eat when you are hungry.* If you decide to follow a specific diet plan, it will be necessary for you to have a total carb gram count in mind every day.

Although the total carbohydrate counts vary, all of the diet plans reviewed in this book suggest that carbohydrates be kept to a minimum. In his book *The Ketogenic Diet*, Lyle McDonald defines a low carbohydrate diet as one that restricts carbohydrates to fewer than 100 grams per day. Dr. Robert Atkins suggests that carbohydrates be kept under 20 grams per day when beginning his low carbohydrate diet plan.

Most of the diet plans stress how easy a low carb diet is. You eat when you are hungry. Period. Just make sure you eat foods that have little or no carbohydrate content.

As you can see from Table 5–1, a typical daily vegetarian menu might not include the essential proteins and fats found in a low-carb diet. A typical daily low-fat menu might also severely restrict these same foods.

TABLE 5–1. DAILY CARB GRAM TOTALS FOR DIFFERENT LIFESTYLES

NON-DIETER	Carb count
Breakfast	
Cinnamon swirl Danish	55g
Orange juice	28g
Coffee w/ cream & sugar	4g
Lunch	
Cheeseburger	31g
French fries	49g
Large soda	35g
Brownie	48g
Snack	
Potato chips	60g
Soda	35g
Dinner	
Fried chicken	15g
Baked potato	50g
Corn on the cob	23g
White bread roll	16g
Carrot cake	40g
TOTAL	**489g**

LOW-FAT	Carb count
Breakfast	
Blueberry muffin	40g
Low-fat latte	3g
Banana	27g
Lunch	
Turkey sandwich	40g
Apple	21g
Raspberry ice tea	37g
Snack	
Energy bar	45g
Apple juice	36g
Dinner	
Pasta primavera	45g
Green salad w/ croutons and low-fat dressing	10g
French bread	45g
White wine	10g
Low-fat yogurt & cookies	49g
TOTAL	**408g**

VEGETARIAN	Carb count
Breakfast	
Raisin bran muffin	38g
Herbal tea	0g
Orange	21g
Lunch	
Hummus & veggies on pita	95g
Papaya nectar	34g
Snack	
Grapes	16g
Peanuts	12g
Dinner	
Veggie lasagna	40g
Garlic bread	28g
Mixed green salad w/ oil and vinegar	3g
White wine	10g
Lemon sorbet	31g
Oatmeal raisin cookies	24g
TOTAL	**352g**

LOW-CARB	Carb count
Breakfast	
Cheese omelet w/ ham	7g
Decaf coffee	0g
Lunch	
Hamburger patty w/ cheese and bacon, no bun	0g
Salad w/ blue cheese dressing	5g
Herbal ice tea	0g
Snack	
Cheese and celery	3g
Decaf sugar-free cola	0g
Dinner	
Filet mignon	0g
Asparagus w/ butter sauce	2g
Mixed green salad w/ parmesan dressing	5g
Low-carb cheesecake	2g
Decaf coffee	0g
TOTAL	**24g**

Good News / Bad News

That brings us to the good news and the bad news. Unlike low fat diets, you will not eliminate foods that contain essential proteins and fats, such as meat, fish and poultry. All of these foods have a zero carbohydrate count (see Table 5–2). You are encouraged to include them in every meal.

This is probably contrary to all the dieting advice you've ever received. Don't be surprised when your friends and family question your sanity. Just give them a copy of this book and let them judge for themselves. The science is there to support this way of eating, so don't allow yourself to be discouraged or dissuaded by others.

More good news is that you are allowed cheese and cream, as well as other dairy products. This is because they contain less than one gram of carbohydrate per ounce. Milk, on the other hand, has 11 carbohydrate grams per cup, so it is not generally allowed. So, instead of sorbet and low-fat cookies for dessert, indulge with blackberries and a dollop of artificially-sweetened real whipped cream. Let's not forget eggs. A low carbohydrate lifestyle allows you to eat them at every breakfast if you choose.

Still more good news is that you no longer have to eliminate foods such as regular salad dressings and mayonnaise (see Table 5–2). Make sure that none of the products you purchase are low fat or include sugar. If you use bottled varieties of dressings, remember to check the label for carbohydrate content. Some are very high because of added sugar and occasionally balsamic vinegar.

Now for the bad news. Low carbohydrate gurus have differing ideas about the suitability of including fruit in your diet. Some say avoid fruit altogether and some say you can eat all fruit but in *very limited amounts*. It is important to be aware of the carbohydrate gram content of the fruit you eat and make sure that you do not exceed your target total carbohydrate gram count for each day.

Most of the gurus suggest the fruits listed in Table 5–3 because they have relatively low carbohydrate content. Be very careful when adding fruit to your daily meal plan. If you find yourself at a plateau, too much fruit may be the culprit.

Now for the really bad news. Grains (cereals, breads, pasta, etc.)

TABLE 5-2.   FOODS THAT CONTAIN 1 CARBOHYDRATE GRAM OR LESS

MEATS (0 carbs)

bacon	ham	lamb	rabbit
beef	hamburger	pastrami	sausages
corned beef	hot dogs	pork	venison

FOWL (0 carbs))

capon	duck	pheasant	turkey
chicken	goose	quail	
cornish hen	partridge	squab	

FISH AND SHELLFISH (0 carbs)

bass	flounder	perch	smelt
bluefish	haddock	salmon	sole
calamari	halibut	sardines	sturgeon
clams	lobster	scallops	swordfish
cod	monkfish	scrod	trout
crabmeat	oysters	shrimp	tuna

DAIRY (1 gram or less per ounce)

cottage cheese	cream cheese	hard cheese	yogurt (some)
cream	eggs	sour cream	

FATS / OILS / DRESSINGS (0 carbs)

butter	olive oil	soybean oil	walnut oil
corn oil	safflower oil	sunflower oil	
mayonnaise	sesame oil	vegetable oil	

are the most controversial foods among low carb advocates. Because of the high carbohydrate content of grains, most low carb writers require that grains be very limited or even totally eliminated. A few are more generous. No matter which low carb diet plan you choose, all recommend only whole grain products.

Likewise, because of their high starch content, root vegetables like carrots and potatoes are not allowed on low carb diets. See Table 5–4 for a list of vegetables that can be usually included in a low carbohydrate diet.

TABLE 5–3. FRUITS WITH LOW CARBOHYDRATE CONTENT

apricots	1/2 cup	<9g
blackberries	1/2 cup	<10g
blueberries	1/2 cup	10g
cantaloupe	1/2 cup	<7g
cherries	12 grams	9g
coconut, fresh	1 oz.	<5g
peaches	1/2 cup	<10g
plums	1/2 cup	<11g
raspberries	1/2 cup	7g
strawberries	1/2 cup	<6g

Planning Ahead

With carbohydrate-counting in mind, you'll find it helpful to have some tools at hand to assist you. A book that lists foods and their carbohydrate values is essential. If you have access to the internet, there are online sites and software that can also help.

A low carb diet does require that you be prepared. Weekly menu planning and a carefully prepared shopping list are essential to successful low carbohydrate dieting. Shopping is simplified, however. Nearly all of the interior aisles of your supermarket can be avoided. You'll find yourself concentrating on the exterior aisles that contain dairy, meat, fish, poultry and produce. This is because meat, fish, poultry and most dairy have zero or low carbohydrates. So no more walking up and down all the aisles and reading labels for fat content.

Boredom is another aspect of any diet that is important to address. It's easy to find yourself in a rut eating the same old thing every day, simply out of convenience. This pattern can easily lead to boredom which inevitably leads to cheating. To avoid this pattern, it's a good idea to invest in one or two low carb cookbooks. Fran McCullough's *Low Carb Cookbook* (reviewed in chapter 9) is a good one to have on hand. Check with your local bookstore for other titles or search online. There are loads of great recipes for low carb entrees, snacks and desserts, including home-made ice-cream. Remember, it's the sugar, not the cream that has the carbs. Table 5-5 lists foods that can help to add zest and variety to a low carb diet.

TABLE 5–4   VEGETABLES WITH LOW CARBOHYDRATE CONTENT

alfalfa sprouts	1 cup	4g
artichoke hearts	1/2 cup	<10g
arugula	1 oz.	1g
avocado	1 medium	12g
bamboo shoots	1/2 cup	<2g
beet greens	1/2 cup	<1g
broccoli	1/2 cup	<4g
Brussels sprouts	1/2 cup	<7g
cabbage	1/2 cup	<4g
cauliflower	1/2 cup	<3g
celery	1/2 cup	<3g
chard	1/2 cup	<4g
collard greens	1/2 cup	<4g
cucumber	1/2 cup	<2g
eggplant	1/2 cup	<4g
endive	1/2 cup	<1g
kale	1/2 cup	<4g
kohlrabi	1/2 cup	<6g
leeks	1/2 cup	4g
lettuce	1-1/2 cups	1g
mushroom	1/2 cup	<2g
okra	1/2 cup	<6g
onions	1/2 cup	<7g
parsley	1/2 cup	<2g
peppers, sweet	1/2 cup	<4g
pumpkin	1/2 cup	6g
radishes	1/2 cup	2g
rhubarb	1/2 cup	<3g
scallions	1/2 cup	<4g
snow peas	1/2 cup	<6g
spaghetti squash	1/2 cup	5g
spinach	1/2 cup	<4g
string beans	1/2 cup	<5g
tomatoes	1/2 cup	<5g
turnips	1/2 cup	<6g
turnip greens	1/2 cup	3g
watercress	1/2 cup	<1g
wax beans	1/2 cup	<4g
zucchini squash	1/2 cup	<5g

TABLE 5–5   CARBOHYDRATE CONTENT OF MISCELLANEOUS FOODS

almonds, dried	1 oz.	6g
almond butter	1 tbsp	<3g
capers	1 tsp	<1g
dill pickles	1 oz	1g
garlic	1 clove	1g
green olives	10	<1g
herbs	1 tbsp	<1g
horseradish	1 tsp	<1g
mustard	1 tsp	<1g
pecans	1 oz.	<5g
peanuts	1/2 cup	<14g
peanut butter	2 tbsp	5g
pepper	1 tsp	<1g
pork rinds	1/2 oz	0g
salt	1 tsp	0g
spices	1 tsp	0g
sugar-free Jello	1 cup	<1g
Tabasco sauce	1 tbsp	0g
tofu	1/2 cup	<3g
walnuts	1/4 cup	3g

Like anything else in life, once you've established your routine, you'll find this way of eating to be easy. And, after a couple of days, you'll begin to notice that your cravings for bread, pasta and sweets will either diminish or disappear completely.

All diet plans recommend that you drink at least eight glasses of water per day. Other beverages should be limited to those that are sugar- and caffeine-free. Some diet plans say you can include some alcoholic beverages. However, wine and beer are usually high in carbohydrates.

It is generally recommended that prepared or pre-packaged foods be avoided or scrutinized for carbohydrate content. These foods frequently contain hidden sugars as well as preservatives and additives, some of which prevent absorption of necessary nutrients.

VEGETARIANS

For many years a vegetarian diet was considered perhaps the healthiest way to eat. However, some current research has shown that most vegetarians are deficient in both protein and fat. Most of the books reviewed (in chapters 7 through 9) address the vegetarian diet and how to make it healthier by adding more fat and protein.

The Carbohydrate Addict's LifeSpan Program™ (reviewed in chapter 7) offers a week's worth of meal plans including meat, fish and fowl alternatives that are available at supermarkets and health-food stores. Addresses and phone numbers of the manufacturers are given along with fifteen recipes.

In *The Zone,* (reviewed in chapter 9) Dr. Barry Sears compares a vegetarian diet, a "recommended healthy" diet, and the American Diabetes Association diet with *The Zone* diet. Dr. Sears clearly illustrates the differences between them, focusing on the ratio of carbohydrate, protein and fat in each. A few recipes and some vegetarian protein suggestions are offered as well.

Dr. Diana Schwarzbein, in *The Schwarzbein Principle* (reviewed in chapter 8), presents the most comprehensive advice for vegetarians who are interested in eating a more balanced diet. She says ". . . I never discourage anyone from eating a vegetarian diet. I discourage eating a bad vegetarian diet. . . ." Dr. Schwarzbein offers four weeks of vegetarian meal plans and has also co-authored a cookbook for vegetarians: *The Schwarzbein Principle Vegetarian Cookbook.*

CHAPTER 6

The Healthy Low Carb Lifestyle

Do, or do not. There is no try.

Yoda

THE DREADED "E" WORD

Just as there are different opinions about diets, there are controversial opinions about what kind of exercise is best for us. Proponents of low carbohydrate eating do seem to agree on two things, however. First: exercise—now matter what kind—is an important part of cardiovascular and psychological health and should be done consistently. Second: most people will *not* lose weight, even with a moderate amount of exercise, if their body continues to produce high levels of insulin. This explains why you can exercise on a low fat diet and not lose that spare tire.

Endorphins

For people who are overweight and out-of-shape, depression and lethargy are familiar territories. However, it is important to know

*It is essential that you consult your physician
before beginning any exercise program.*

that exercise—even moderate exercise—will cause you to you feel better. Why? Because of endorphins.

In 1975, Dr. Hanz Kosterlitz and Dr. John Hughes made an important discovery. They found that the brain produces morphine-like chemicals which, when stimulated, create a sense of well-being. These morphine-like substances are called endorphins. Exercise is one thing that signals the brain to release endorphins. Researchers have since found that endorphins are responsible for:

- pain control
- relieving stress
- enhancing our immune system
- Improving blood circulation

Meditation, laughter, sexual activity, and a good mental attitude can also signal the brain to release endorphins. So, endorphins can be released when you watch a funny movie. (A good idea when you're recovering from an illness.) Quiet, focused meditation can also release endorphins. However, researchers have proven that nothing produces larger amounts of these mighty endorphins than vigorous aerobic activity.

Aerobic Exercise

The term "aerobic exercise" means activity done *with oxygen*. Such activity must involve the same large muscle group for at least 15 to 20 minutes while maintaining 60 to 85 percent of your maximum heart rate. Aerobic activities include walking, jogging, running, cycling, swimming, cross-country skiing, jumping rope, skating, rowing, dancing, or climbing stairs.

To sustain any of these activities you would use the same large muscle group and it would be necessary for you to breathe deeply and regularly. It would also be necessary for your heart to maintain 60 to 85 percent of its maximum rate. This 60 to 85 percent range is called your target heart range (THR).

You can figure your THR by first obtaining your maximum heart rate, or MHR. To do that, subtract your age from 220. The resulting number is your MHR. Let's say you're 40 years old. Your MHR would be 180 [220 – 40 = 180]. To find your THR, multiply your MHR by 60 percent [180 x 60% = 108] and again by 85 percent [180 x 85% = 153]. These resulting two numbers are your THR. The target heart range for someone who is forty is 108–153.

Anaerobic Exercise

While aerobic exercise means an activity that requires oxygen, anaerobic exercise is the opposite. Obviously, all activity requires oxygen, but anaerobic activities do not require a steady intake of oxygen. Anaerobic activities are those which generally keep you from gasping for breath. For instance, an athlete running a 25-yard dash would not normally have to take a breath during the run.

Some anaerobic activities are weight lifting, golf, tennis, manual labor, jai-alai, football, hockey, rugby and gymnastics. Although exercise professionals categorize certain activities as either aerobic or anaerobic, it is possible to perform some exercises in ways that can make them either. For instance, walking is generally considered aerobic. However, walking the dog and allowing him to stop and sniff every 25 feet isn't.

Perhaps the most important anaerobic exercise is weight lifting. More properly called resistance training, it builds lean body mass. When lean body mass is increased, your metabolism speeds up. When your metabolism speeds up, you burn fat more efficiently. If you need to lose body fat, an increased metabolism will speed up that process.

Human Growth Hormone

Exercise is one way of releasing human growth hormone (HGH). Often called the master hormone, HGH regulates muscle-to-fat ratio and causes the body to burn fat instead of glucose for energy. It also boosts the immune system, prompts healing, enlivens libido, enhances brain function and helps to maintain internal organs and skin.

As we age, HGH release decreases. However, strenuous exercise, especially weight or resistance training, significantly increases the release of HGH. Shapely muscles, reduced body fat and stronger bones associated with resistance training are largely due to the release of HGH. As little as ten minutes of intense resistance work, two or three times per week, can have a noticeable effect.

It's important to note here that the release of HGH can be effected by diet as well. When bloodstream insulin levels are high the body slows down or stops HGH release altogether. A carbohydrate snack before bedtime will slow the release of the HGH that the body normally releases when we first enter deep sleep. Similarly, a carbohydrate snack to increase energy prior to resistance training will block HGH release normally associated with this activity. So will consuming a high carbohydrate sports drink *during* the workout.

Exercise Success

Most exercise professionals suggest three to five aerobic workouts each week. If you haven't been exercising then start out with 10–15 minutes each day, adding five minutes every other workout until you have reached 30 minutes for each workout. Sixty minutes is the maximum amount of time you should spend for a workout.

Start slowly. Those words should be posted everywhere in your house—on the refrigerator, bathroom mirror, the front door, even in the car—as a constant reminder. There's no benefit in enrolling in an intermediate aerobics class if you haven't been participating in any sort of regimented activity in some time. You'll become discouraged, injured or both and then be right back on the sofa, wondering why you even bothered.

Choose an activity that you enjoy. What's the point of jogging four times a week if you hate every minute of it?

Keep a diary. You will be amazed at how recording your daily activity can be an inspiration. If you skip your activity for a day or a week, be honest with yourself, write down the reasons why and then get moving again. Don't beat yourself up for missing a class or not walking because of bad weather. Get out there the next day, congratulate yourself and record your accomplishment in your journal.

The most important part of an exercise program is warming up prior to any activity and cooling down afterward. Stretching and warming up should be part of every exercise routine, before and after. This prepares the muscles for strenuous exercise and helps to prevent injury to tight, unused muscles. Warming up prepares the heart in the same way. It tells your heart you are getting ready to give it a workout and allows it to build slowly.

In the process of getting fit you will be losing weight and building muscle mass. Muscle is heavier than fat so don't get discouraged if you step on the scales and it hasn't budged a pound. Chances are you can now button those old jeans.

There are many good books on the market which will guide you through any exercise program you choose. Just make sure that the program you choose is designed for your level of fitness and offers a good stretching routine. Don't pick a plan designed for the intermediate or advanced athlete if you haven't exercised for years. Choose a plan that fits not only your fitness level but your lifestyle as well. It's your body, your choice. Make it a good one.

THE IMPORTANCE OF WATER

Whatever your diet, all the experts agree that water is an essential part of any weight loss program. Bottled, boiled, filtered, strained or right out of the tap, enough is almost always not enough.

Water is second only to oxygen as essential for life. Without water you could perish in as little as three days. A consistent intake of water replenishes your body's cooling system which is designed to help you survive extreme heat and elevated body temperatures. Water is necessary for the digestion and absorption of food. It flushes waste from your body, helps you maintain proper muscle tone, and supplies oxygen and nutrients to your cells.

It is estimated that water comprises 60–70 percent of our body weight. On average, females have a lower percentage of water in their body because females tend to have more body fat. Leaner body, more water. More fat, less water. Simple.

Water and Weight Loss

Almost without exception all of the low carbohydrate diet plans advocate drinking at least eight glasses of water daily. This is because when you burn fat (without consuming large amounts of carbohydrates) some of the fat may be burned incompletely. As mentioned earlier, these fat by-products are called ketones. Your body will burn these or dispose of them in your urine, stool or breath. The more water you drink the more urine you produce, and, thus, the more incompletely burned fat—or ketones—are passed through the urine.

How Much Water Do You Really Need?

If you incorporate exercise into your weight loss program, you will need to increase your water intake in order to keep your tissues hydrated. Eight glasses a day may not be enough if you increase your activity level. It is important to know that once you *notice* you are thirsty your body has *already* become somewhat dehydrated.

One suggestion is to record your water consumption for a couple of days, to make sure you know how much you are drinking. If, throughout your normal routine, you are not getting the required eight glasses a day, you'll know that you'll have to increase your intake. An easy way to do this is to keep that bottle or glass filled at your desk, in your car, or on your bike. Remember, every time you drink water, you are flushing toxins—including fat—from your body.

About Those Diet Drinks. . . .

Few diet plans advocate substituting diet drinks for water. There is much controversy surrounding sugar-free and/or diet drinks containing artificial sweeteners. Many researchers believe that the consumption of these drinks could prevent weight loss by signalling the pancreas to produce insulin simply because of their sweet taste. In other words, diet colas *may be* keeping you fat.

In his book *Your Body's Many Cries For Water*, Dr. Fereydoon Batmanghelidj suggests that artificial sweeteners—being 180 times as sweet as sugar—are responsible for fat storage, increased hunger and a myriad of illnesses. His book is a must read for anyone who doubts the value of drinking eight glasses of water daily. Batmanghelidj suggests that the current health care crisis is because we are not aware when the human body is thirsty for water.

Caffeinated Beverages

Have you ever heard someone say that they are addicted to caffeine? They probably are. The National Clearing House for Drug and Alcohol Information classifies caffeine as addictive because withdrawal produces symptoms. However, The World Health Organization says that "There is no evidence whatsoever that caffeine use has even remotely comparable physical and social consequences which are associated with serious drugs of abuse." Then the American Psychiatric Association says there is such a thing as caffeine intoxication, a condition caused by "high caffeine intake."

Caffeine is a naturally occurring substance found in the leaves, seeds or fruits of at least 63 plant species worldwide. The most commonly known sources are coffee and cocoa beans, kola nuts and tea leaves. After entering the bloodstream caffeine does a number of things. It stimulates the brain and blood pressure and pulse rate are increased. There is also an increase in the production of stomach acid and a release of fatty acids in the blood. Anxiety and insomnia are just two of the psychological side effects of the consumption of caffeine.

Everybody has an opinion on caffeine, including the authors of all the diet plan books reviewed in chapters 7 through 9. Some authors suggest that caffeine should be eliminated totally because there are people who are so sensitive that even a small amount may raise insulin levels. Other writers feel that limited amounts of caffeine have no effect on weight loss whatsoever. The predominant sentiment, however, is moderation in all things.

If you think you can't live without your cup of java in the morning, you may want to think again. If you're doing everything else right and you still can't lose those extra pounds, a number of low carbohydrate diet authors suggest you look at your caffeine consumption as a possible culprit.

NUTRITIONAL SUPPLEMENTS

It is generally agreed among health care professionals that the best way to get vitamins and minerals is from foods grown in soil rich in nutrients. The majority of those same health care professionals would also tell you that it is a pretty difficult thing to do these days. Most of the fruits and vegetables we buy at our local supermarket have been grown in soil depleted of essential nutrients and fertilized with chemicals.

We know that some vitamins and minerals aid in protecting us from certain diseases, but there is much disagreement among the experts about which are essential and which are not. The low carb authors reviewed in this book have varying opinions as well.

The only diet plan among those reviewed in chapters 7–9 that makes no recommendation whatsoever is *Sugar Busters!*™ The authors merely alert the reader to the possibility of sugar in pill coatings or filler. *The Zone* author Dr. Barry Sears believes it is not necessary to take supplements if you consume a completely balanced macronutrient diet—in other words, *The Zone*.

Certainly the most comprehensive recommendations come from Dr. Atkins. He has even formulated his own line of supplements that he calls Targeted Nutrition. This, he says, allows him to prescribe for specific nutritional needs. To summarize his recommendations here would be impossible—they take up eight pages in the *New Diet Revolution*.

Atkins believes strongly in the power of nutrients to improve general health. Toward that end he has written a book that focuses almost exclusively on this issue: *Dr. Atkins' Vita-Nutrient Solution: Nature's Answer to Drugs*. If you fear that a low carb diet would not offer you enough nutrients, either of Atkins' books will give you excellent advice on nutritional supplements.

CHAPTER 7

Four Groundbreaking Low Carb Diet Books Reviewed

The recent interest in low carbohydrate diets began with Dr. Atkins' initial publication some twenty years ago. Since that time he has published several other books, and other low carb weight-loss researchers have followed in his wake. The books reviewed in this chapter have all achieved popularity and have dedicated disciples. They differ slightly in their approach, degree, and technique, but all stress the value of restricting carbohydrates in your diet.

DR. ATKINS' *NEW* DIET REVOLUTION / Revised and Updated

Robert C. Atkins, M.D.

348 pps., $21.95, ISBN 0-87131-886-5

Published by M. Evans and Company, Inc., 216 East 49th Street, New York, NY 10017

Twenty years ago when Dr. Atkins published his very controversial best seller, *Dr. Atkins' Diet Revolution*, it was denounced by medical authorities for its low-carbohydrate, high-calorie regimen. Since that time, Atkins has expanded his ideas in *Dr. Atkins' New*

Diet Revolution. The book has new information as well as many case histories that serve to document his findings. He claims success with 25,000 overweight patients, a fact that lends credence to his theories.

Readers will notice almost immediately that Atkins takes a very defensive stance throughout. For instance, he makes sure to define ketosis as "Benign Dietary Ketosis" and not simply ketosis. Speaking of ketosis he says it

> is one of life's charmed gifts . . . as delightful as sex and sunshine. . . .

No doubt this defensive position is the result of two decades of criticism from the pro-establishment researchers who insist that low fat diets are the only way to lose weight. Also much in evidence is the frequent mention of the line of nutritional supplements sold under his name.

One of the most outstanding things about *Dr. Atkins' New Diet Revolution*, however, is that it presents an enormous amount of technical information in a way that can be easily understood. For instance, the information presented on insulin is very comprehensive yet *interesting*. Now there's a concept!

The author doesn't waste much time setting out the reasons his diet plan works. Briefly:

• It creates more fat mobilization than any other diet.
• Keeps the dieter from becoming hungry.
• It's the easiest diet for weight loss maintenance.
• It is a high energy diet.
• It is a healthy diet that helps to correct diet-related disorders.
• It helps to control insulin.

Atkins makes it very clear that not everyone loses weight with ease. He says that those with a less-than-average degree of metabolic resistance will lose anywhere from 8 to 15 pounds in two weeks and those with an average level of resistance, somewhat less.

Atkins defines and describes four stages for his diet program:

• The *14-Day Induction*
• *Ongoing Weight Loss* diet

- *Pre-Maintenance* diet
- *Maintenance* diet

In the second chapter, *What This Book Will Reveal To You,* Atkins carefully details exactly what the reader should expect from his diet plan. In list format, he addresses the diet experience, the weight, health, food and family changes the dieter may expect, as well as how to maintain the weight loss.

For those readers who are still confused about whether or not they really need a ketogenic diet, Atkins profiles his typical obese patient, asking the reader to answer some simple questions about eating habits, health, mood swings and so on. After taking this short test you should be able to determine if the Atkins diet plan is right for you.

Atkins is very thorough, presenting research and scientific fact to support his claims. There is a good deal of information to help the reader support this low carbohydrate diet. For instance, he discusses the controversy that low carbohydrate diets have generated, and he strives—through the presentation of easy-to-understand research—to document his dietary claims. Also included is a chart that outlines the pre-Atkins and post-Atkins calorie intake of a patient who was able to lose fifty pounds in three months. He consumed only 201 fewer calories per day on the Atkins plan.

Atkins outlines steps to take before starting the *14-Day Induction* diet. These include the cessation of any unnecessary medications, a medical checkup that includes extensive blood tests and, most importantly, a five-hour glucose-tolerance test (GTT) with insulin levels. After you've accomplished all this, you are ready to start the *Induction* diet. The rules are:

- no more than 20 grams of carbohydrates a day
- eat until you are satisfied
- you must not even touch any food that is not allowed
- foods that combine protein with carbohydrates or fat with carbohydrates are not allowed
- follow the *Carbohydrate Gram Counter* at the back of the book very closely

These rules are followed by a two-page list of foods that are allowed as well as some helpful tips. Allowed foods are all meat, all fish, all fowl, all shellfish, all eggs, almost all cheeses, loads of vegetables, any beverage without caffeine (sorry, no alcohol) and plenty of essential oils such as olive, canola, and walnut and, oh yes, butter and cream. No fruit or bread.

A dieters typical daily menu on Atkins' *Induction* diet might look something like this:

Breakfast bacon and cheese omelet
Lunch salad with dressing, roast beef with cheese (no bun)
Dinner lobster cocktail, beef consomme, steak, salad with
      dressing

Two other important aspects of the *Induction* diet are discussed—supplements and lipolysis testing strips. Atkins recommends vitamins and minerals for this 14-day diet. A more comprehensive, long term regimen is given later. Lipolysis testing strips are used to measure the degree of ketosis/lipolysis in urine. Atkins believes they can be an important aid to losing weight on this diet plan. For those dieters who are not losing weight as fast as they would like or who are simply stalled, lipolysis strips may help to answer some questions.

Atkins provides a short quiz to help readers evaluate lipolysis test results. He also suggests that certain blood tests be taken again to get a clear picture of just how his diet has effected important health issues (like cholesterol).

A discussion of "diet-related disorder syndrome" is presented. This phrase was coined by Atkins to describe symptoms sometimes evidenced by his patients that related to their diet (unstable blood glucose, food intolerances and yeast syndrome). He also discusses the benefits of restricting carbohydrate consumption for people with heart disease. And he makes nutritional support recommendations for those people who, even with the diet, have difficulty achieving satisfactory blood lipid levels.

After dieters finish the *14-Day Induction* diet, it's time to move on to the *Ongoing Weight-Loss* diet. With the help of a few charts Atkins maintains that weight loss can continue if the dieter keeps these two basic principles in mind:

• Fewer carbohydrates consumed means greater weight loss
• Carbohydrate consumption can be controlled

A typical day on Atkins' *Ongoing Weight Loss* diet might look like this:

Breakfast eggs Benedict, 3 oz. tomato juice, 2 slices toasted
     diet bread with butter
Lunch Tuna salad in half avocado, clear soup, beverage
Dinner beef tartare, lobster in drawn butter, Caesar salad
     (without croutons), half-cup strawberries in cream

For the person that he describes as the "metabolically resistant" dieter, Atkins has developed the *Fat Fast*. Without a doubt, it is sure to raise some eyebrows. It consists of 1,000 calories, ninety percent of which are from fat. The *Fat Fast* is not designed for people who want to lose a few pounds fast but for those who have difficulty achieving success by just restricting carbohydrate intake. Atkins suggests that metabolic resistance may be the result of several things, including anti-arthritic medications and antidepressants, steroids and diuretics or oral antidiabetics. Other culprits might be hormone imbalance or an underactive thyroid. Blood tests can answer these questions.

During a *Fat Fast,* the day's food intake should be broken down into four small "feedings" of 250 calories each or five of 200 calories each. He provides examples of what these "meals" might contain.

Atkins' *Pre-Maintenance* diet is designed for those who have only five to ten pounds left to lose. Although the low-carb regimen can be relaxed somewhat, the author cautions that adding carbo-hydrates that weren't allowed previously should be done carefully and slowly.

The end of Dr. Atkins' program isn't really the end. The *Main-tenance* diet is the way one eats after weight loss is achieved. A typ-ical *Maintenance* daily menu might include

Breakfast one cup strawberries with small amount of
     whipped cream, western omelet with cheese, diet toast
     with butter
Lunch salad with cold lobster, goat cheese and egg, rasp-
     berries with dollop of whipped cream
Dinner cream of chicken soup, beef Stroganoff, one cup
     Brussels sprouts, vanilla ice cream with fresh blueberries,
     glass of dry wine or two wine spritzers

Atkins offers some good tips and answers some questions to help keep the dieter on the right path. The importance of exercise and nutritional supplements round out the body of this groundbreaking diet book, along with 43 recipes by Graham Newbould, the man Atkins calls his "master low-carbohydrate chef." Newbould was formerly chef to the Prince and Princess of Wales. *Lobster Soup, Cheese Pancakes, Chicken Curry, Walnut Butter Cookies* and *Chocolate Truffles* are just a few of the recipes included.

THE CARBOHYDRATE ADDICT'S LIFESPAN PROGRAM™: A Personalized Plan for Becoming Slim, Fit, & Healthy in Your 40s, 50s, 60s & Beyond.

Richard F. Heller, M.S., Ph.D.
Rachael F. Heller, M.A., M.Ph., Ph.D.

475 pps., $14.95, ISBN 0-452-27838-4

Published by Plume, an imprint of Dutton Signet, a member of Penguin Putnam Inc. 375 Hudson Street, New York, NY 10014.

This has become one of the most popular diet plans in the country since the Hellers appeared on the Oprah Winfrey Show in September, 1999. The popularity of their diet program has skyrocketed so much that finding a copy of their book may be more difficult than staying on their plan.

Despite the fact that people on their diet often characterize it as low carb, the Hellers were adamant on the Oprah Winfrey Show that theirs is not a low carb diet. Low carb diets release ketones, and they consider ketones dangerous. Nevertheless, because so many people consider it a low carb diet, and because it is a diet that *restricts* carbohydrates, it will be reviewed here.

Do you get light headed, tired or cranky after a meal?
Have you gained weight easier as you've aged?
Does stress make you hungry?
Do you include some kind of sugar with most of your meals?

If you are over 40 and have answered "yes" to one or more of these questions, Drs. Rachel and Richard Heller believe you may be experiencing a physical addiction to carbohydrates.

This book is based on their popular 1991 *Carbohydrate Addict's Diet*™. The Hellers, both former research scientists and professors at Mt. Sinai School of Medicine, have since refined their ideas and recommendations. Having lost and kept off a total of 200 pounds between them, the authors carefully and clearly outline how easy it is to suppress food cravings by keeping insulin levels in check. Starting with stories of their own personal weight loss struggles, they lay out a "Basic Plan" with only three guidelines:

1. *For two of your three daily meals—and when snacking— eat only those foods which will reduce cravings.* A list of "Craving-Reducing Foods" (all low carbohydrate) are helpful in determining just what foods are allowed.

2. *The third meal of the day will be a "Reward Meal*™*."* This meal should consist of equal parts high carbohydrate foods, protein and Craving-Reducing vegetables. Thus, this meal could include potatoes and dessert, as long as the portion sizes are equal to those of the accompanying protein and low-carb vegetables. The authors offer a list of acceptable high carbohydrate foods.

3. *The Reward Meal*™ *must be completed within sixty minutes.* The Hellers explain the reasoning for this thoroughly. In summary, they say that the time limitation is necessary because insulin is released in two waves when carbohydrates are eaten. The first release is governed by the amount of carbohydrates consumed during the previous twelve to twenty hours. The second release depends upon the amount of carbohydrates consumed at that particular meal. By eating the Reward Meal™ within sixty minutes, they reason, insulin levels are kept low because the meal is completed "before the second wave of insulin release has reached its peak."

The authors have used several patient stories to draw attention to facts they feel are significant. Most importantly, however, they have included several charts, one of which will help the reader to determine if they are a carbohydrate addict or merely succumbing to an occasional indulgence.

Readers can also take a simple fifteen-question test to determine the extent of their addiction. The Hellers maintain that by following the instructions carefully readers can find out whether or not they are carbohydrate-addicted as accurately as (and far cheaper than) with a glucose tolerance test. The test scores are broken down into four categories: Doubtful Addiction, Mild Addiction, Moderate Addiction and Strong Addiction.

Once a level of addiction is established, the Hellers define what they call "triggers," These are things that may cause weight gain, weight retention or that effect one's inability to lose weight. Identified as triggers are carbohydrates, sugar substitutes, MSG and fourteen over-the-counter medications such as antacids and diuretics. All can stimulate the release of too much insulin. Besides these "triggers," events such as surgery, menopause and just plain old age can be a cause of excess insulin.

The book then goes on to address all of the immune system disorders—heart disease, gout, diabetes and some forms of cancer—that research has shown to be effected by elevated insulin levels.

After two weeks of the Basic Plan with its daily two Crave-Reducing Meals and one Reward Meal™, now what? The authors offer nine "Options" which they encourage the dieter to add to the Basic Plan at their discretion. Simple things like taking a chromium supplement, reducing caffeine and sugar substitutes or just making an effort to reduce stress in your life.

Speaking of sugar substitutes, the Hellers are among the few authors who recommend low carb dieters stay away from what most of us feel is our only real extravagance. Although they offer no specific scientific studies, their clinical experience has shown that our beloved sugar substitutes cause an excess release of insulin which, in turn, cause the well known cravings and weight gain. They say that "if it tastes sweet, your body thinks it is getting sugar."

Another interesting aspect of this diet plan is that the Hellers do not stress exercise. They suggest that using mild activity to reduce insulin levels is more important than "burning" calories. This certainly is good news for those who don't have the time or the motivation to "feel the burn" seven days a week. They offer charts that break down all types of activity into three categories: light, moderate and vigorous. They suggest that the reader choose one and and do it consistently as little as 15 minutes a day, three times a week. The focus is that no matter what activity you choose, be consistent.

One thing the authors do stress, however, is the importance of weighing yourself and doing it accurately. In fact, they feel it is so important that they discuss the merits extensively, explain how to average one week's weight, and have designed charts to make it easier to keep track of the disappearing pounds.

A day eating the *Carbohydrate Addict's Lifespan Program*™ way might look like this:

> *Craving-Reducing Breakfast* Cheese and mushroom omelet, sausage (cannot contain sugar), iced or hot coffee or tea
> *Craving-Reducing Lunch* Grilled hamburger, steamed asparagus, salad with vinegar and oil dressing
> *Reward Meal*™ *Dinner* Salad with all the fixings, steamed cauliflower with cheese sauce, filet mignon, rolls or bread with butter, chocolate cake with ice cream and strawberries, coffee

Before coming to an extensive array of recipes, vegetarians will find a week's worth of meal plans and three pages of meat, fish and poultry alternatives as well. And, those on low-fat, low-salt or other restricted diets will find many ways to combine the *Carbohydrate Addicts LifeSpan Program*™ with their own.

PROTEIN POWER

Michael R. Eades, M.D.
Mary Dan Eades, M.D.

429 pps., $6.99, ISBN 0-553-57475-2

Published by Bantam Books, 1540 Broadway, New York, NY 10036

First published in 1996, this book was written by two doctors who share a weight-loss and family medicine practice. After developing the diet they experimented on themselves and then suggested it for their patients. In the ten years they have been treating patients with this program, the Eades claim they "have never had a negative outcome." Although they say that constant refining and research is what makes *Protein Power* so successful, the Eades acknowledge that this diet may not work for everyone because of what they call "biochemical individuality."

The *Protein Power* plan is divided into two phases, one for those who need to lose twenty or more percent of their body weight, and the other for those who simply want to recompose their muscle-to-fat ratio. The diet is a way of eating that is not only nutritionally complete but even allows for some of those things that are missed on many other low carb diets, such as the moderate consumption of alcohol.

One appealing aspect of the book is its brief summaries. Called "The Bottom Line," this helpful tool assists the reader in understanding the scientific data that is presented throughout the book. For readers who don't have the time or the interest, skipping right to these summaries would probably supply most of the information needed to follow this diet, although naturally this is neither a good idea nor recommended.

Several charts throughout the book outline the role of insulin and glucagon, compute body fat percentage, and compare various kinds of carbohydrates. Did you know that one-quarter of a very small potato equals one caramel candy which in turn equals one-seventh of a Milky Way bar? And on and on. There are also four "Protein Equivalency" charts, followed by eleven pages that list the carbohydrate content of most fruits, vegetables, breads, cereals and grains.

Conveniently, the authors also present "The Program in a Nutshell" that is designed to help the reader put together all of the information previously presented:

- calculate your protein needs and the number of carbohydrates appropriate for either their "Intervention" or "Phase II" diet (unlike Atkins, only non-fiber carbohydrate grams are counted.)
- consume 25 grams of fiber every day

- choose healthy fats
- don't be afraid to snack
- drink lots of water
- if you choose to drink a glass of wine a day be sure to count the carbs
- make sure you take a high quality vitamin supplement
- no sugar and starches
- don't forget to exercise

As with a food journal, the Eades also offer a daily meal outline which they recommend be filled out each day. They include a restaurant dining guide as well as an informative question and answer section.

Protein Power presents more detailed medical information than many of the other low carbohydrate books. The authors offer a medical history test to help assess the risk of insulin-related disorders and suggest a battery of blood tests that they explain in great detail. They also thoroughly address the importance of vitamins and minerals, suggest appropriate supplements and make product suggestions.

A day following the *Protein Power* plan might look like this:

Breakfast Ham and cheese omelet, half-cup fresh melon, one slice light bread toast with butter

Lunch Grilled chicken, salad with oil vinaigrette, one fresh peach

Snacks (one of the following, if desired and allowed) 1 oz. macadamia nuts, one-half orange, one-half tomato, half-cup dry red wine; coffee, tea, or mineral water

Dinner Grilled shrimp, two cups salad with oil vinaigrette, broccoli, strawberries with cream

About 75 appealing recipes—including some yummy deserts for those who can't help themselves—will keep this diet from becoming monotonous. How does *Espresso Ice Cream with Cinnamon* and *Irish Lace Cookies* sound? Or perhaps *Chocolate Chip Cheesecake*?

While the focus of the book is on the science of nutrition and a balanced diet, the importance of exercise is not neglected. True to form, the Eades discuss, in detail, the importance of exercise and how it not only will help weight loss but will increase the production of human growth hormone. Calling it the *youth hormone,* the authors list the factors that stimulate its release. These include:

- Lowered blood glucose levels
- Increased blood protein levels
- Low carbohydrate diet
- Fasting
- Increased protein intake
- Plenty of the right kind of exercise

They also list some factors that inhibit human growth hormone release:

- High blood glucose levels
- Being overweight

All of these factors are discussed in fascinating detail along with some great suggestions on how to get started on your way to becoming healthier and stronger.

The Eades take great pains to outline the science of their diet plan and detail just how this way of eating will help to eliminate fat and aid the healing of immune system disorders. They also explain the importance of *eicosanoids,* a group of at least 100 hormone-like substances that control nearly all physiological actions such as blood pressure, blood clotting, pain and fever response, and the sleep/wake cycle. Food, the authors say, plays a very large role in the balance of eicosanoids. Informative as it is, for those who can't wade through the scientific data, the authors take the time to sum it up succinctly.

Wrapping up this detailed diet plan Drs. Michael and Mary Dan Eades present some interesting historical facts, starting with the ancient Egyptians (yes, there are obese mummies!) and end with a few pages of helpful "Sources and Resources."

SUGAR BUSTERS!™ Cut Sugar To Trim Fat

H. Leighton Steward
Sam S. Andrews, M.D.
Morrison C. Bethea, M.D.
Luis A. Balart, M.D.

272 pps., $23.95, ISBN 0-345-42558-8

Published by The Ballantine Publishing Group, a Division of Random House, Inc., New York. www.randomhouse.com

Sugar Busters!™ is one of the easiest to understand of all the low carb diet books. Written by a cardiovascular surgeon, an endocrinologist, a gastroenterologist and the former CEO of a Fortune 500 company, *Sugar Busters!*™ sold over 100,000 copies by word of mouth when it was first published independently as a softcover in 1995. It is now available in an updated hardcover edition.

It is important to note that unlike the older softcover, the newer hardcover includes a fourteen-day eating plan, 82 pages of recipes, a question and answer section, and a helpful index. If you simply want an overview of the diet and feel confident enough to construct your own eating plan and recipes then by all means get the paperback. If exotic recipes such as *Filet de Boeuf Nature Marchand de Vin* or *Crabmeat Yvonne* sound enticing, then pick up the hardcover edition.

The authors strive to relate the essence of their findings in the *Introduction* that helps to make the information on insulin, diabetes and hypoglycemia easier to follow. The basis for the *Sugar Busters!*™ way of eating is in its title—a low-sugar diet, consisting of fresh meats, most vegetables and fruits, some dairy, whole-grain breads and pasta, brown rice and nuts.

Carbohydrates are not counted here. Importance is placed on the glycemic index. The glycemic index indicates the ability of a specific food to raise blood sugar levels. To aid the reader, the authors offer easy-to-read glycemic index charts separating grains, breads and cereals from fruits, vegetables and dairy. They have rated foods in each group either high, moderate or low. For instance, white bread is high (95), rye grain is low (35); a baked potato is high (95), kidney beans are low (30); watermelon is high (70), fresh apricots are low (10); and, premium ice cream is high (60), plain yogurt is low (15).

This is what a day of eating the *Sugar Busters!*™ way might be like:

Breakfast Oatmeal with milk, orange or grapefruit juice
Lunch Turkey and cheese on whole grain bread with lettuce, dill pickle, light mayonnaise
Dinner Grilled lamb chops, mushrooms sauteed in olive oil, spinach salad, lima beans

The history of sugar production is provided with graphs that chart per person sugar consumption from 500 A.D. onward. Also interesting is a discussion devoted to diet myths such as "fat and weight gain" and "alcohol is always bad for you" (for those who refuse to give up that glass of red wine with dinner).

Most interesting, however, is the discussion on calories and weight loss. The authors state that most calorie research studies were "performed decades ago." According to *their* research, these studies were not verified or reviewed in the same manner as research results are today. Also, they say, after a number of overeating studies were tabulated, it was determined that calculating the number of calories consumed was not enough to predict weight gain or loss. But, as can be confirmed by many of today's most popular diets—all low fat—counting calories is still widely accepted.

Diabetics may be interested to know that the authors offer extensive information on how *Sugar Busters!*™ can work for them. One charts compares obesity with the likelihood of developing diabetes within ten years. Food group tables are presented as helpful guides for shopping and planning meals, and there is a short table of acceptable substitutions for foods such as the beloved baked potato, corn and white bread.

The authors also compare a typical "balanced American diet" with a recommended *Sugar Busters!*™ diet. For example, a typical "balanced" breakfast of juice with sweet roll, cereal or toast and jelly along with caffeinated coffee or tea is designed to make your insulin skyrocket. The *Sugar Busters!*™ alternative breakfast might begin with a piece of fruit consumed one-half hour before the rest of the meal. The remainder of the meal might consist of two eggs; sugarless sausage; one slice of whole-grain toast with butter and decaf coffee or tea.

The authors wind up this easy-to-follow diet plan with eight pages of questions and answers, a glossary, references, and a helpful index. If you are looking for a diet plan that is based on the glycemic index, not on counting carbs and want your information straight and simple, this is the diet book for you.

CHAPTER 8

Seven More Effective Low Carb Diet Books Reviewed

These books offer significant variation in their approach to low carb dieting. All are important and informative. While not as well known as those in the preceding chapter, they deserve wider recognition and can serve as valuable resources.

NEANDERTHIN / Eat Like a Caveman to Achieve a Lean, Strong, Healthy Body

Ray Audette with Troy Gilchrist

204 pps., $23.95, ISBN 0-312-24338-3

Published by St. Martin's Press, 575 Fifth Ave., New York, NY 10010

The premise of what is certainly one of the most unique low carb books on the market is that our bodies need only those foods that can be found in nature. Another way to express the basic tenet of this book is to point out that obesity is practically unknown in the wild among animals or humans. In the wild, animals and humans do not eat factory-processed foods.

Written by a former rheumatoid arthritis and diabetes sufferer, *NeanderThin* is based on the natural diet of the Paleolithic hunter-gatherer. Ray Audette has formulated a diet plan that includes only those things that would be edible if we were stripped of all technology and armed with only a rock or a sharp stick.

NeanderThin was first published in 1995 and is now in its fourth edition. In a foreword, Dr. Michael R. Eades (author of *Protein Power*) says that the *NeanderThin* diet is very similar to the eating plan that he has advocated for many years.

Few of us subsist on what we hunt and kill, nor, for the most part, do we find our vegetables, fruits, berries and nuts in the wild. Nevertheless, Audette suggests we emulate as best we can, the diet of people who do hunt and forage. Even if the average reader finds such a regime daunting, this book is highly recommended. Audette's unique commentary and perspective on contemporary diet is well-worth reading. Audette pointedly reminds us that the way we eat has been drastically transformed from what was once a diet based on natural food to one of factory-processed foods. This, he maintains, is unnatural and unhealthy.

Audette provides a fascinating history of how our contemporary ideas about food and diet have come about. He describes his search to cure his rheumatoid arthritis and diabetes, one that ultimately led him to formulate *NeanderThin's* natural way of eating. He outlines, with great clarity, the function of the immune system and the various immune system diseases that have blossomed since the advent of technologically-produced foods. He suggests—startlingly—that 95 percent of people in developed countries will die of immune systems diseases such as Krone's disease, multiple sclerosis, Alzheimer's, and many forms of cancer and lupus. He also describes how these diseases are linked to obesity and how obesity is linked to the low fat, low protein, high carbohydrate diet prevalent today.

Audette issues his own "Ten Commandments," divided equally between foods that should be eaten and foods that are never to be eaten. *Never,* he says, should we eat grains, beans, potatoes, dairy or sugar. We *must* eat meats, fruits, vegetables, nuts and berries. Alcohol and coffee is strictly forbidden.

The rules are so simple, it would be difficult to make a mistake about what to look for at your supermarket—the modern human's savanna. Also offered are tips such as what steps to take before starting, how to include your spouse and friends, and what to order when dining in restaurants. Audette is firm in his belief that it is not possible to be a vegetarian on this diet.

For those who are concerned about adapting to such a radical change in diet, Audette gives the reader menu suggestions and a sample diary that describes what he might have during a one week period. This includes breakfasts (eggs with vegetables cooked in olive oil, uncured bacon), lunches (chicken, salad, strawberries), dinners (shrimp, raw oysters, tuna steak and salad), and snacks (beef jerky, fruit, nuts).

Forty pages of recipes are presented, including several soups, salads, entrees and desserts. He also provides the reader with instructions on how to make what he considers a *NeanderThin* diet staple: *pemmican*. A combination of dried meat and beef fat, Audette describes it as a high energy "snack for the modern hunter-gatherer."

There are several pages of questions and answers and an incredibly comprehensive bibliography. Even if you're not thinking about using *NeanderThin* to lose weight you might want to pick up a copy just for its fascinating, well-organized perspective on the ills of the average contemporary diet.

DR. TONY PERRONE'S BODY-FAT BREAKTHRU / 10 Personalized Fat Fighting Plans for Mega-Health

Tony Perrone, Ph.D. with Mark Laska

284 pps., $24, ISBN 0-06-039274-6

Published by ReganBooks, an imprint of HarperCollins Publishers, Inc., 10 East 53rd Street, New York, NY 10022

Known as "Hollywood's body fat expert" because of clients such as Demi Moore, Bruce Willis and Denzel Washington, Dr. Perrone offers not just one but ten diet plans. Perrone believes that because each person's metabolism is unique there should be a diet plan to address those individual needs. It is not weight that we want to lose, he says, but rather it's body fat that needs to be trimmed.

To determine which plan is best for you, you must first answer ten questionnaires. According to the author, once you have answered all the questions, the plan with the largest number of "yes" answers is the most effective plan for you.

The plans vary in complexity and duration. At the conclusion of some of the plans, you are instructed to answer the questionnaires again. The assumption is that your metabolism may have changed and another plan may now be more appropriate for you. The process continues until you reach your goal.

All of the plans have been structured for specific metabolic problems. They include his "Insulin Buster Plan," the "Unlimited Protein and Vegetables Plan," a "50/30/20 Plan," and so on. The author even offers a "7-Day Quick Fix" for those dieters with only seven pounds of fat to lose. He does caution, however, that this plan should be used only for seven days and no more since it consists of five meals a day, four of which are protein shakes only.

A Ph.D. in clinical nutrition, Perrone simply and clearly presents important information about insulin, fat and protein to support his diet plans. Also included is information on exercise and nutrients that he says may accelerate weight loss. Some helpful hints about such things as alcoholic beverages and scales plus 41 interesting recipes round off this unique approach to weight loss.

Some of the plans are complicated and require some thought and planning. Perrone begins each plan with comments on that plan's ease of use, how hard it will be to dine out, the rate of fat reduction, the duration and how much energy you can expect to have. Having selected a plan through the questionnaire method, it is assumed that your metabolism is performing in a certain way, and Perrone explains what that is and how it can be corrected.

This unique approach to what is essentially low carb dieting is valuable for its variety and individuality. It may not be appropriate for readers who want simple answers and solutions to their weight problem. It will be valuable to individuals who want to closely monitor and understand the process of their fat loss.

THE SCHWARZBEIN PRINCIPLE /
The truth about losing weight, being healthy and feeling younger

Diana Schwarzbein, M.D.
Nancy Deville

365 pps., $12.95, ISBN 1-55874-680-3

Published by Health Communications, Inc., 3201 S.W. 15th Street, Deerfield Beach, FL 33442-8190

This is one of the most comprehensive, informative and balanced diet plans available today. If you are interested in losing weight and maintaining your health, this is the plan for you.

The founder of the Endocrinology Institute of Santa Barbara, Dr. Schwarzbein approached diet with an eye toward how the food we eat affects our hormones. She gives us several examples of patients who dramatically changed their lives by changing their diets. This is a very helpful tool. You just might find your own life mirrored in one of these amazing examples.

Schwarzbein carefully and clearly lays out the reasons why low fat diets haven't worked and she cites important research to substantiate her claims. She also addresses the difficulty of losing body fat on a low calorie diet. Her message is so clear and concise that most people will have no trouble understanding the science.

Dr. Schwarzbein is among those who think that ketones are dangerous. She believes that the way to lose body fat is to "first heal your metabolism." This, she says, is done by eating all the right foods in the proper amounts.

Vegetarians should take note that Schwarzbein expresses her concern that most vegetarians do not consume enough protein. Because insufficient protein can lead to elevated insulin levels and enumerable health problems, she offers advice on how to eat a more balanced diet without consuming animal products, and provides four weeks' worth of vegetarian meal plans.

This diet plan is packed with eye-opening information and many helpful hints. Do yourself a favor and read this one.

EAT FAT, LOSE WEIGHT / How the Right Fats Can Make You Thin for Life

**Ann Louise Gittleman, M.S., C.N.S.
with Dina R. Nunziato, C.S.W.**

154 pps., $14.95, ISBN 0-87983-966-X

**Published by Keats Publishing, a division of NTC/
Contemporary Publishing Group, Inc., 4255 West Touhy
Avenue, Lincolnwood, IL 60646-1975**

Unlike most of the other diet plans, Gittleman's main focus is on the importance of fat in our diet and how two decades of low fat eating has created a nation of overweight Americans.

There is plenty of good information about omega oils and the role they play in a healthy diet. The author supplies the standard insulin and protein facts necessary to the understanding of why low fat diets don't work.

She bases her diet plan not on carbohydrate grams but on the glycemic index and offers a list of foods with their glycemic rating. This means that more grains are allowed on this diet plan than on most other low carbohydrate plans.

This is a very simple and easy-to-follow plan with a few good hints, supplement suggestions and ideas on how to stock your pantry and fridge. Although not as comprehensive as some of the more popular diet plans, if you don't have the time or the interest to go through them, then this is the one for you.

CHARLES HUNT'S DIET EVOLUTION™ / "Eat Fat and Get Fit!"

Charles Hunt

196 pps., $19.95, ISBN 0-9630377-1-4

**Published by Maximum Human Potential Productions,
311 N. Robertson Blvd., Suite 130, Beverly Hills, CA 90211.
Orders: 1-877-988-4668.**

With a foreword by Drs. Michael and Mary Dan Eades, authors of

Protein Power, Charles Hunt's plan is based on the hunter-gatherer diet. He claims that throughout history whenever grains were the central focus of our diet, the health of humanity has been compromised.

This diet plan is very similar to that of Atkins, although Hunt doesn't present it in as scientific a manner. However, the straight what-you-really-need-to-know facts are offered. According to the author, eggs, cheese, meat, fish, fowl, most vegetables and berries with cream for dessert are what it takes to get healthy and lose weight. He supplies us with 233 recipes to keep us from getting bored. Even one for rattlesnake. Yum.

A former investigative reporter, Hunt cites loads of research to support his claims that a hunter-gatherer diet is the only healthy diet. His diet plan is a very personal one. Hunt himself spent many years fighting a weight problem (years of yo-yo dieting) and ill health, including a heart attack and blood sugar problems. Hunt, now healthy and in fantastic shape (as is evidenced by the nude profile of the author on the book's cover) is sharing his hard-earned information with us. An enjoyable and informative read and a good low carb diet plan.

STARCH MADNESS / Paleolithic Nutrition for Today

Richard L. Heinrich

155 pps. ISBN 1-57733-027-7

Published by Blue Dolphin Publishing, PO Box 8, Nevada City, CA 95959. Orders: 1-800-643-0765.

With a forward written by *The Zone* author Barry Sears, this diet plan offers, as its cover suggests, "healthy eating guidelines that really work."

This book is not so much a diet plan as a diet education. Eleven of the 14 chapters begin with citations of one, two or more publications about diet, nutrition or well-being. The works cited serve as the basis of each chapter's theme. Heinrich reviews and comments on the ideas and research that are found in each of the works.

Overall, he finds the most sensible approach to low carb diets is one that is based on monitoring the glycemic index of foods. Such an approach allows for the inclusion of some carbohydrates in the diet, including low-glycemic grains, fruits and vegetables. Filled with an impressive amount of research data as well as the author's personal experiences, Heinrich's plan is similar to *The Zone*. In fact, Heinrich devotes considerable attention to the benefits of *The Zone*.

This is an intelligent and well-written book. With some information on exercise, water and the many benefits of Vitamin C, this plan is appropriate for dieters who are willing to delve into the science of low carbohydrate diets.

THE KETOGENIC DIET / A Complete Guide for the Dieter and Practitioner

Lyle McDonald

323 pps., $29.95, no ISBN #.

Published by Lyle McDonald, 8885 Research Blvd., Apt. 1169, Austin, TX 78758

Lyle McDonald defines a ketogenic diet as one that ". . . restricts carbohydrates below a certain level (generally 100 grams a day)."

This "Guide" is without a doubt the most comprehensive reference available for those interested in understanding how low carbohydrate diets work. While it is appropriate for the dieter, health care professional and bodybuilder, its emphasis is on the relationship of low carb diets and exercise. It offers fully referenced information on everything from the physiology of ketosis to carefully structured exercise programs for all levels.

McDonald makes the point that while low carb diets are effective when combined with moderate exercise, individuals who engage in high-intensity exercise will need to incorporate carbohydrates into their diet. He outlines how this can be done without "disrupting the effects of ketosis." He offers two different diet plans that incorporate carbohydrates. One, the "targeted ketogenic diet" or TKD, allows for carbohydrates to be eaten near the period of exercise. The other, "cyclical ketogenic diet" or CKD, alternates periods of low and high carbohydrate intake.

This guide stands alone among all the other diet plans because of its technical detail. If you are likely to be discouraged by page after page of scientific data or just don't have the time or interest, this is not for you. However, if you are the kind of person who wants to know *in detail* how a low carbohydrate diet works along with exercise, this reference guide will be an invaluable resource for you.

CHAPTER 9

Three "Almost Low Carb Diet Books" Reviewed

Strictly speaking, the books reviewed in this chapter are not low carb diet books. One provides information on low carb cooking. The other two are included because they are often considered by many people to be low carb diet plans. They restrict refined carbohydrates, but allow for a wider range of complex carbs.

THE ZONE / A Dietary Road Map

Barry Sears, Ph.D. with Bill Lawren

286 pps., $23, ISBN 0-06-039150-2

Published by ReganBooks, an imprint of HarperCollins Publishers, 10 East 53rd Street,New York, NY 10022.

Based on Sears' Nobel Prize-winning research in dietary control of hormonal responses and cancer treatment, *The Zone* was a leader in the pack of books asking us to look in a totally different way at how we eat.

Although *The Zone* cannot accurately be described as a low carb diet, it does limit the amount of carbohydrates consumed. More importantly, Sears presents an immense amount of scientific information substantiating his ideas about how diet effects hormones, and how hormones effect body weight and health. Sears focuses on eicosanoids, which he calls superhormones. Sears and the Eades (*Protein Power*) are the only low carb authors reviewed in this book to discuss the importance of eicosanoids. They are so little discussed in general that he says that your physician is unlikely to be familiar with them. He maintains that eicosanoids are

> the most powerful biological agents known to man. Control eicosanoids, and you'll open the door to the Zone.

According to Sears, eicosanoids control the body's hormonal systems and nearly all of the body's vital functions. The point of *The Zone* is that if you follow the diet, you will control the proper balance of good and bad eicosanoids in the body. *The Zone* is all about balance.

Although it has a large following, some people may find the plan difficult because of the way it is structured. Meals must be perfectly balanced following the author's "macronutrient food block" charts. Each meal consists of the appropriate number of protein, carbohydrate and fat blocks.

What are blocks? A protein block, for example, consists of seven grams of protein. The number of daily protein blocks you require is figured on the basis of your lean body mass times your activity level. Charts are provided to assist you in these calculations. Other food blocks are figured in the same way, however their gram weight differs. Fat blocks are 1.5 grams each for example. The total number of blocks consumed is spread out over three meals and two snacks.

The bottom line on *The Zone* is that it is a serious book for people who are serious about their health as well as losing weight. It is a great resource for those who want to know more about how food effects hormone production.

40-30-30 FAT BURNING NUTRITION:
The Dietary Hormonal Connection to Permanent Weight Loss and Better Health

Joyce and Gene Daoust

116 pps., $16.95, ISBN 1-56912-086-2

Published by Wharton Publishing, Del Mar, CA

Weight-loss and sports nutritionists Joyce and Gene Daust say that there are no good or bad foods—what is important is to achieve the correct balance of foods in your diet.

The Dausts were once sales reps for a leading amino acid manufacturer and as such became technical advisors to their clients: doctors, gym personnel, health food stores, etc. In 1991 they began to work with Dr. Barry Sears (*The Zone* author). They reviewed numerous amino acid profiles and were struck by the high incidence of amino acid deficiencies, even in people who ate adequate protein. They concluded that Sear's diet recommendations of 40 percent carbohydrate, 30 percent protein and 30 percent good fat made sense. They tried it themselves (Gene Daust was a bodybuilder) and both saw positive results by reducing their intake of carbohydrates.

Their basic dietary recommendations, therefore, are similar to *The Zone*. *40-30-30 Fat Burning Nutrition* doesn't contain the technical detail of other diet plans, but it is well organized and simple to follow. The book guides the reader through the how's and why's with the help of many easy-to-read charts such as:

- a chart of high-quality protein foods
- several pages devoted to the nutritional values of the most common foods
- a glycemic index chart demonstrating that rice cakes increase blood glucose five times faster than a plum!

Included with the charts and graphs are highlighted boxes that summarizes important information. This may be helpful to readers who like their information neatly condensed and easily available.

Just by flipping through the pages it's simple to access important details by focusing on the highlighted boxes.

Based on the glycemic index, this plan cannot accurately be described as a low carbohydrate diet. As in *The Zone*, 40 percent of its total nutrition comes from high-fiber carbohydrates such as grapefruit, peaches and other low glycemic fruits, most vegetables, and whole wheat breads, beans, nuts and seeds.

Because they are sports nutritionists, the Daousts offer some excellent information on exercise and fitness. They suggest that "carb loading" before, during or right after exercise inhibits the release of glucagon and human growth hormone. This forces the body to burn glucose instead of stored fat. They believe their *40-30-30 Fat-Burning Nutrition* prevents this by keeping blood sugar levels stable and also by releasing more glucagon.

Besides hypoglycemia, Type II diabetes, high blood pressure and high cholesterol, the Daousts believe their diet plan helps boost the immune system, relieve premenstrual syndrome symptoms, lift depression, stabilize mood swings, and curb sleep disorders. They actually suggest that it can help those individuals who have difficulty *gaining* weight. There are three pages devoted to those who prefer a vegetarian diet as well as a week's worth of suggested meals along with a few recipes.

In order to use the plan the reader must first locate their particular body type on the "Meal Planner Conversion Chart." This chart specifies activity level and weight for both women and men. Once your body type is identified (you are either an A, B, C or D) then you follow the *40-30-30 Fat-Burning Nutrition* chart that is designed to eliminate any guesswork about just how many grams of carbohydrate, protein and fat you need at each meal. For instance, if you are a "B," you would require 20g of carbohydrate, 15g of protein and 6g of fat at breakfast. Sounds complicated, but actually they have made it quite easy to follow.

The authors present a week's worth of meals for each of the four body types, all very organized and easy to follow. Also included is one week's worth of what the Daousts call "Fat-Flush Meals." These meals are designed for those who wish to "accelerate fat loss to near genetic maximum rates." The Fat-Flush Meals can be used for several weeks at a time. In Fat-Flush Meals, high glycemic carbohydrates have been eliminated in favor of lots of high-fiber foods and low- to medium-carb foods.

"Tips and Hints," a six-page food value guide, a discussion on restaurant eating, a chart listing the nutritional composition of prepared foods and a short chapter on supplements bring to an end this simple yet informative diet plan.

THE LOW-CARB COOKBOOK / The Complete Guide to the Healthy Low-Carbohydrate Lifestyle: With over 250 delicious recipes . . . .

Frank McCullough

384 pps., $22.95, ISBN 0-7868-6273-4

Published by Hyperion, 114 Fifth Avenue, New York, NY 10011

Although not a diet plan of its own, this is an important book to have on hand if you plan on maintaining a low carb lifestyle. McCullough, like a lot of the other low carbohydrate authors, struggled with her weight and health problems. A cookbook editor, she was the first editor of *Protein Power* by Michael and Mary Dan Eades.

Their ideas made sense to her, and she became a convert, losing 60 pounds by incorporating their principles into her cooking. As a food afficionado, however, she saw the need for a good low carbohydrate cookbook, and this is it. As the Eades point out in their foreword to this book, when *their* book came out there were hundreds of titles on low fat cooking but not a single one on low carb cooking. The *Low-Carb Cookbook* is the first *good* cookbook available for the low carb lifestyle.

Included are over 300 interesting recipes along with menus to follow for a low carb Thanksgiving, Christmas and New Year's Eve. Other menus, like "Mexican Dinner" and "Middle Eastern Dinner" will help to keep you from becoming bored with the same old fare.

McCullough prefaces her recipes with some low carbohydrate science in addition to offering some very helpful hints. Information on artificial sweeteners, how to deal with plateaus, and how to stock your kitchen are but a few. Each recipe includes a per-serving protein, fat and carbohydrate count.

If you want to make the jump to a low carb diet but are hesitant because of what seems to be a lack of variety, you must acquire this book. It will help you see that there are numerous ways to prepare a variety of flavorful low carbohydrate meals.

Foods Allowed on Six Different Diet Plans

By now you should have a fairly good idea which diet plan is best for you. To further aid your decision process, this chart outlines foods allowed on six different diet plans. Naturally, because sugar is eliminated from a low carb diet, this chart does not include foods such as cookies, candy, cakes, etc.

This is intended as a general guide only. Consult the specific diet plan books for more complete food lists. For instance, almost *any* food would be allowed in a Reward Meal™ on the *Carbohydrate Addict's Lifespan Program™*. Note also that this list does not allow for some sugar-free substitute foods. For example, *Atkins'* allows ice cream if it is *homemade* with a sugar substitute.

key: ■ = allowed
       □ = allowed in limited amounts
       × = not allowed

	PROTEIN POWER	ATKINS' INDUCTION DIET	CARBOHYDRATE ADDICT'S™	THE ZONE	SUGAR-BUSTERS™	NEANDER-THIN
MEATS / FOWL / FISH	■	■	■	□	■	■
VEGETABLES broccoli	□	□	□	□	□	■
carrots	□	×	□	□	×	■
cauliflower	□	□	□	□	□	■
corn	□	×	□	□	×	×
cucumber	□	□	□	□	□	■
green beans	□	□	□	□	□	×
lettuce	□	□	□	□	□	■

Foods Allowed on Six Different Diet Plans (cont.)

	Protein Power	Atkins' Induction Diet	Carbohydrate Addict's™	The Zone	Sugar-Busters™	Neander-Thin
Vegetables (con't)						
peas	□	×	□	□	□	×
potatoes	□	×	□	□	×	×
tomatoes	□	×	□	□	×	×
Fruit						
apple	□	×	□	□	□	■
avocado	□	■	□	×	□	■
banana	□	×	□	□	×	■
blueberries	□	×	□	□	□	■
cherries	□	×	□	□	□	■
melon	□	×	□	□	□	■
orange	□	×	□	□	□	■
peach	□	×	□	□	□	■
pear	□	×	□	□	□	■
plum	□	×	□	□	□	■
strawberries	□	×	□	□	□	■
Dairy						
butter	□	■	□	□	□	×
cheese, hard	×	■	□	□	□	×
cheese, cottage	×	■	□	×	□	×
cheese, low fat cottage	□	×	□	□	×	×
cream, heavy	×	■	□	×	□	×
cream, half & half	×	×	□	×	×	×
eggs	×	■	□	□	□	×
ice cream	×	×	□	×	×	×
milk, low fat	×	×	□	□	×	×
milk, whole	×	×	□	×	□	×
yogurt	×	×	□	□	□	×
Grains						
bread, whole grain	□	×	□	□	□	×
crackers, high-fiber	□	×	□	□	□	×
oatmeal	□	×	□	□	□	×
pasta, whole grain	□	×	□	□	□	×
rice, brown	□	×	□	□	□	×

Frequently Asked Questions

The important thing is not to stop questioning.
—Albert Einstein

Q *Okay, I'd like to try this. How do I get started?*

A First and most importantly, see your doctor and get an accu-
rate assessment of your overall health. This might include a wide
range of blood tests, although not all of the low carb diet book
authors believe this is necessary.

Next, make a decision about which diet plan book most
appeals to you based on the reviews in chapters 7 through 9. Then
go to the library or bookstore and read it for yourself. See if it suits
your needs. Be realistic. Choose one that you feel can fit into your
lifestyle and that you won't abandon within a week or two. Keep
in mind that all of the diet plan books discussed here emphasize
low carbohydrate consumption as a way of life, not just a way to
lose weight.

It is also helpful to have a friend or family member on the same
or similar plan. This way you can support each other and do your
meal planning and grocery shopping together. Eventually you will
be able to go to the mall together when all your old clothes need
to be replaced with smaller sizes!

Q *Do I absolutely have to go to a doctor for blood tests?*

A Nearly all of the low carbohydrate plans recommend seeing your doctor for even the minimum tests. Not only is this just plain good sense, it will give you a baseline from which you can follow your progress. Knowing what your cholesterol and blood sugar figures are before you start restricting carbohydrates will be clear evidence of the effectiveness of a low carb diet.

Q *How would this way of eating change my life?*

A Well, for starters, if you're not good at receiving compliments then don't embark on a low carbohydrate diet! It won't take friends and family long to notice you've become trimmer. You'll hear comments along the line of "What have you been doing?" or "Gee, you look great!"

More importantly, you'll also have a lot of extra energy and improve your overall health. Low carbohydrate diets are not difficult to follow. You just have to re-think the way you eat.

Q *A friend went on a low carb diet for six months, lost a lot of weight and then put it all back on again when she returned to a low-fat diet. Will this happen to me?*

A First of all, a low carb diet is not just a diet, it's a lifestyle. When maintained, it keeps excess fat off.

Secondly, yes, you probably would gain back the pounds you lost if you switched back to a low fat diet. This is because when you revert to low fat, you start up your fat storing machine. On a low fat diet you produce excess amounts of insulin that will convert carbohydrates to stored fat.

Q *Do I have to eat like this for the rest of my life?*

A All of the low carbohydrate diet plans stress the importance of maintaining a lifetime of *sensible* eating.

This means not falling back on the constant consumption of refined carbohydrates. That's what got you in trouble in the first place. Remember, what's most important is to keep insulin from spiking and dropping. That's what makes you hungry and makes you crave those bags of cheese doodles and sugary soda.

So be realistic. If you've reached your goal weight and you want an occasional snack, go ahead and treat yourself. There's nothing that makes you want to abandon a diet faster than feeling deprived. Just remember that too many of these treats will put you right back on the extra insulin-producing track—which means packing on those unwanted extra pounds.

Q *Can I still eat in restaurants?*

A Virtually all of the low carb diet books reviewed here give ideas for eating in restaurants. Even fast food can be acceptable if you follow some simple rules: don't eat the bread, watch the salad dressing (no low fat!) and skip the french fries and colas.

Believe it or not you can even eat at your favorite little Italian bistro if the sight of everyone around you eating pasta and bread doesn't bring you to tears. For example, you can order chicken in wine and garlic sauce with a salad, or fresh grilled fish with sauteed vegetables.

Q *What about alcohol?*

A The jury still seems to be out on this question. *Sugar Busters!*™ maintains that it's okay to have a glass of red wine with dinner, although the authors are quick to point out that alcohol will not *help* you lose weight. *Protein Power* suggests that a glass of dry wine helps to *lower* insulin levels and the authors cite several studies to back that up.

If you decide that *Carbohydrate Addict's*™ is the diet plan for you, then you may have a glass or two of your favorite alcoholic beverage during your Reward Meal™. Dr. Atkins recommends only hard alcoholic beverages be consumed and then only during the maintenance phase of his diet. And finally, the author of *NeanderThin* suggests that the "preferred method of intoxication" for hunter-gatherers is ingesting herbs and not alcohol.

Q *I'm a vegetarian. Can I still eat a low carb diet?*

A Of all the low carb diet books discussed, only *NeanderThin* states emphatically that you cannot be a vegetarian and eat low carb. All the others offer meal plan suggestions along with special tips for vegetarians. However, most are careful to point out that getting enough protein is a difficult thing to do if you are not consuming *animal* protein. If you are a committed vegetarian, *The Schwarzbein Principle* has some very good suggestions for maintaining a healthy low carb vegetarian diet. Dr. Schwarzbein has also written a cookbook for vegetarians.

Q *I'm overweight but my family is not. Is a low carb diet healthy for all of us?*

A Alsolutely. The benefits that you notice—increased energy, etc.—will be felt by your family too. You will lose your excess fat, and they will maintain their svelte figures. They may even notice an increase in their muscle-to-fat body ratio.

More seriously, an astounding proportion of Americans die each year from immune system diseases, most of which are now thought to be related to a rise in insulin brought on by the consumption of large amounts of refined carbohydrates. A low carb diet may help to reduce your family's risk of succumbing to auto-immune diseases.

Q *How long will it take me to lose weight on any of these diets?*

A You'll start losing the first week no matter what diet plan you choose. From there on it really depends on the plan. For instance, *Carbohydrate Addict's*™ stresses losing slowly, about one- to one-and-a-half pounds a week. With *Atkins* you can lose as much as three to five pounds a week on his *Induction* diet.

Adding excerise—even moderate exercise—to your weight loss regime will also speed up the rate of loss for you.

Also, although it seems unfair, males loose faster than females.

Q *Is this way of eating more expensive?*

A We all know that a box of dried pasta is cheaper than a sirloin steak. No question about it.

However, consider the rewards you will reap from this small investment in your body. Not only will you lose excess fat, you won't be as prone to autoimmune diseases which—if you're looking at the bottom line—are *really* expensive!

Remember also that on a low carb diet your hunger will diminish and you'll eat less. The feeling among most low carb dieters is that the actual cost of food is a bit more, but not as much as you might think.

Q *Is it okay for children to restrict their carbohydrate intake?*

A For overweight children, yes, absolutely. *The Carboydrate Addict's*™ authors Drs. Heller have even written a book on the subject: *Carbohydrate-Addicted Kids*. And Dr. Atkins believes that even obese babies would benefit from a carbohydrate-restricted diet—under the supervision of a pediatrician.

Average, healthy, active children will probably benefit from additional complex carbohydrates (fruits and vegetables). Restricting excess refined carbohydrates is beneficial and something mothers have attempted for generations: "No more cookies!"

Q *Do I absolutely need to exercise?*

A You probably will lose excess weight on a low carb diet even if you don't add extra activity to your schedule. But all of the low carb diet plans advocate some sort of regular exercise program to improve cardiovascular fitness and to improve your overall quality of life. Even moderate exercise will increase your rate of metabolism and promote increased weight loss. And don't forget those important endorphins for an increased sense of well-being!

Q *I've heard you can get halitosis and constipation on a low carb diet. Is that true?*

A Halitosis can occur during ketosis when some ketones are expelled from the body through urine, stool and breath. If your water intake is sufficient, it is thought that a majority of those ketones will be eliminated through your urine and any bad breath effect diminished. Constipation can occur when your diet does not include adequate fiber and water intake.

Q *What can I say to my friends and relatives who think low carb diets are dangerous?*

A There is a tremendous amount of research that supports the benefits of restricting carbohydrates in the diet. Many of the low carb diet book authors have done extensive research of their own before recommending this way of eating to their patients and clients. *The Zone, The Carbohydrate Addict's LifeSpan Program*™, *The Schwarzbein Principle* and *Dr. Atkins' New Diet Revolution* are great for reassuring yourself and your friends and family about the safety of low carbohydrate eating. These authors have collectively researched low carbohydrate diets for many years and have successfully treated thousands of patients.

Bibliography and
Resources

Atkins, Robert C. *Dr. Atkins' New Diet Revolution*. New York: M. Evans and Company, Inc., 1992, 1999.

Atkins, Robert C. *Dr. Atkins' Nutrition Breakthrough*. New York: William Morrow and Company, Inc., 1981.

Audette, Ray. *NeanderThin*. New York: St. Martin's Press,1999.

Batmanghelidj, F. *Your Body's Many Cries For Water: You Are Not Sick You Are Thirsty*. Falls Church, VA: Global Health Solutions, Inc., 1998.

Bernstein, Richard K. *Dr. Bernstein's Diabetes Solution: A Complete Guide to Achieving Normal Blood Sugars*. New York: Little, Brown & Company, 1997.

Cheraskin, E., and W. M. Ringsdorf, Jr., with Arline Brecher. *Psycho-dietetics, Food as the Key to Emotional Health*. Chelsea, MI: Scarborough House, 1974, 1989.

Daoust, Joyce and Gene Daoust. *40-30-30 Fat Burning Nutrition: The Dietary Hormonal Connection to Permanent Weight Loss and Better Health*. Del Mar, CA: Wharton Publishing, 1996.

Dufty, William. *Sugar Blues*. New York: Warner Books, 1975.

Eades, Michael R. and Mary Dan Eades. *Protein Power*. New York: Bantam Books, 1996, 1998.

Eaton, S.B., and S. B. Eaton, III, et al. "An Evolutionary perspective enhances understanding of human nutritional requirements." *Journal of Nutrition*, 126:1732-40, June 1996.

Eaton, S.B., and M. Konner. "Paleolithic nutrition: A consideration of its nature and current implications." *New England Journal of Medicine*, 312:283-89, Jan.31, 1983.

Eaton, S. Boyd, Marjorie Shostak, and Melvin Konner. *The Paleolithic Prescription*. New York: Harper and Row, 1988.

Fredericks, Carlton. *New Low Blood Sugar and You*. New York: Perigee Books/The Berkley Publishing Group, 1985.

Freeman, John M., Millicent T. Kelly, and Jennifer B. Freeman. *The Epilepsy Diet Treatment: An Introduction to The Ketogenic Diet*. New York: Demos Vermande, 1996.

Gittleman, Ann Louise, with Dina R. Nunsiato. *Eat Fat, Lose Weight: the Right Fats Can Make You Thin for Life*. Lincolnwood, IL: Keats Publishing, 1999.

Heinrich, Richard L. *Starch Madness: Paleolithic Nutrition For Today*. Nevada City, CA: Blue Dolphin Publishing, Inc., 1999.

Heller, Richard F., and Rachael F. Heller. *The Carbohydrate Addict's Lifespan Program: A Personalized Plan for Becoming Slim, Fit, & Healthy in Your 40s, 50s, 60s & Beyond*. New York: Penguin Putnam, Inc., 1998.

Heller, Richard F., and Rachael F. Heller. *Carbohydrate-Addicted Kids: Help Your Child or Teen Break Free of Junk Food and Sugar Cravings—for Life!* New York: HarperCollins Publishers, Inc., 1997.

Heller, Richard F., and Rachael F. Heller *Healthy For Life: Reversing the Single Most Important Health Risk Factor of Your Life*. New York: Penguin Books, 1996.

Hunt, Charles. *Charles Hunt's Diet Evolution*™: *"Eat Fat and Get Fit!"*. Beverly Hills, CA: Maximum Human Potential Productions, 1999.

Liberman, Shari and Nancy Bruning. *The Real Vitamin and Mineral Book: Using Supplements for Optimum Health*. Honesdale, PA: Paragon Press, 1997.

McCullough, Frances Monson. *The Low-Carb Cookbook: The Complete Guide to the Healthy Low-Carbohydrate Lifestyle* etc: New York: Hyperion, 1997.

McDonald, Lyle. *The Ketogenic Diet: A Complete Guide for the Dieter and Practitioner.* n.p., 1998.

Netzer, Corinne T. *The Complete Book of Food Counts.* New York: Dell Publishing, 1997.

Perrone, Tony with Mark Laska. *Dr. Tony Perrone's Body-Fat Breakthru: 10 Personalized Fat Fighting Plans for Mega-Health.* New York: Regan Books, an imprint of HarperCollins Publishers, Inc., 1999.

Schwarzbein, Diana and Nancy Deville. *The Schwarzbein Principle: The Truth About Losing Weight, Being Healthy and Feeling Younger.* Deerfield Beach, FL: Health Communications, Inc., 1999.

Sears, Barry with Bill Lawren. *The Zone: A Dietary Road Map.* New York: HarperCollins Publishers, Inc., 1995.

Steward, H. Leighton, et al. *Sugar Busters!™: Cut Sugar to Trim Fat.* New York: The Ballantine Publishing Group, 1998.

INTERNET RESOURCES

Web links can become outdated quickly. Rather than list links here, LowCarb LifeStyles, Inc., the publisher of this book, maintains a website that contains current links to sites

- about low carb diets and experts
- about health and nutrition
- that offer low carb products and services

Information is also provided on subscribing to low carb lists and message boards. Visit

www.LowCarbLifeStyles.com